Advances in
Child Neuropsychology

Advances in
Child Neuropsychology

Edited by

Michael G. Tramontana
Stephen R. Hooper

Michael G. Tramontana
Stephen R. Hooper

Editors

Advances in Child Neuropsychology

Volume 1

With 17 Illustrations

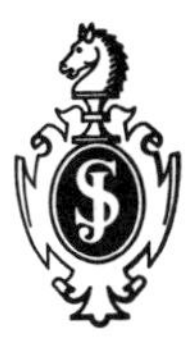

Springer-Verlag
New York Berlin Heidelberg London Paris
Tokyo Hong Kong Barcelona Budapest

Michael G. Tramontana, Ph.D.
Division of Child and Adolescent Psychiatry
Vanderbilt University School of Medicine
Nashville, TN 37212, USA

Stephen R. Hooper, Ph.D.
Department of Psychiatry and the Clinical Center for the Study of Development and Learning
University of North Carolina School of Medicine
Chapel Hill, NC 27514, USA

ISSN: 0940-8606

Printed on acid-free paper.

Production managed by Christin R. Ciresi; Manufacturing supervised by Jacqui Ashri.

Typeset by Best-set Typesetter Ltd., Chai Wan, Hong Kong.
Printed and bound by Edwards Brothers, Inc., Ann Arbor, MI.
Printed in the United States of America.

9 8 7 6 5 4 3 2 1

ISBN 0-387-97611-6 Springer-Verlag New York Berlin Heidelberg
ISBN 3-540-97611-6 Springer-Verlag Berlin Heidelberg New York

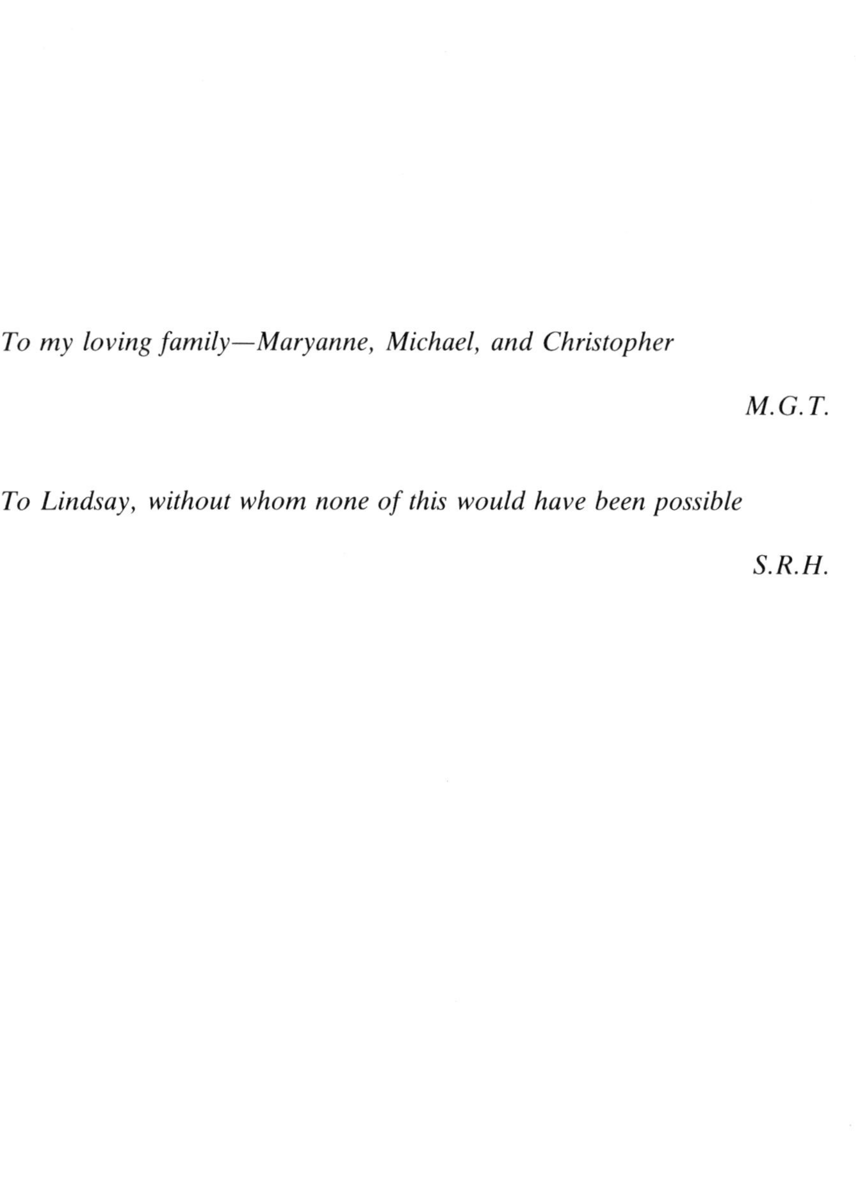

To my loving family—Maryanne, Michael, and Christopher

M.G.T.

To Lindsay, without whom none of this would have been possible

S.R.H.

Foreword

The field of child neuropsychology is still young. It has no obvious birthdate. Hence, we cannot determine its age with the type of chronometric precision for which our scientific hearts may yearn. Nevertheless, one landmark to which we might point in this connection is that the first systematic textbook to appear in this area (i.e., Rourke, Bakker, Fisk, & Strang, 1983) is not yet 10 years old. Be that as it may, activity in the field has been growing steadily, if not by leaps and bounds. Although there is nowhere near the intensity of investigation of children from a neuropsychological standpoint as there is of adults, there have been notable systematic investigations of considerable interest. Some of the more important of these are presented in the current volume.

Intended to provide authoritative reviews of important substantive areas of child neuropsychology, this series begins with a volume that contains just that: reviews of areas as diverse as auditory evoked responses in newborns and the behavioral effects of head trauma in children. Methodological issues, also deemed important by the Editors, are discussed in most of the chapters contained herein. Furthermore, the exemplary lines of programmatic research or application in the field that are deemed to fall within the purview of this series are also represented in this volume. As though this were not sufficient challenge, the Editors also wish to present bridges between research and practice, and to reflect the kind of integrative and innovative work truly indicative of advances in child neuropsychology. This last set of criteria is difficult to meet, but there are glimmerings of such within this volume. Let me be more specific.

In Chapter 1, Molfese presents an incisive review of the literature relating to auditory evoked responses from newborn infants and their predictive validity for language skills measured several years later. This is a particularly intriguing topic, since we are increasingly concerned with the very early prediction of those infants who are most "at risk" for later information processing deficiencies. The demonstrated significance of the methods described in this chapter for the prediction of such deficiencies is impressive, and their clinical significance potentially great.

Two of the chapters in this work have to do with traumatic brain injury in children, but from quite different perspectives. Fennell and Mickel (Chapter 2) provide a substantive review of the research in this area, and Ylvisaker, Szekeres, and Hartwick (Chapter 6) describe a program of assessment and intervention for dealing with the survivors of such trauma. Together these contributions provide a rich source of information regarding the current state-of-the-art in this very important area of neuropsychological inquiry, assessment, and treatment.

As was the case in Chapter 1, Hugdahl (Chapter 5) presents a rather specific review of research dealing with a specific assessment instrument—in this case, dichotic listening. As with the Molfese contribution, we are treated to a review of the relevant studies within this complex area of developmental neuropsychology. In addition, some suggestions are made with respect to the applicability of this technology to the thorny problem of predictive validity.

A specific area of clinical interest in our field—i.e., seizure disorders—is addressed in Chapter 4 by Curley. This chapter includes a very focused review of the literature in this area as well as data from a longitudinal study that was designed to tackle and deal with some of the more difficult issues nascent therein. A reading of this chapter will suggest how very difficult it is to investigate the relevant developmental parameters of even a supposedly circumscribed set of disorders such as these. A fortiori, it will suggest how very difficult it is to recommend with assurance how treatment should proceed, principally because of the paucity of predictive validity data within this—and, for that matter, many—areas of child neuropsychology.

Chapter 3, authored by Taylor, Schatschneider, and Rich, contains a wealth of information. It presents a general and specific review of the literature germane to its focus: it includes data on a longitudinal study of considerable interest; it points to general as well as specific principles that are relevant for assessment and treatment. In a word, it is a contribution to the volume that contains most, if not all, of the characteristics sought by the Editors.

As this cursory review indicates, the contributors to this volume have done what they have been asked to do. They have provided the types of incisive reviews of important topics and/or exemplary lines of programmatic research and application that bode well for the future of this fledgling field. Where appropriate to do so, they have spelled out some of the assessment and treatment implications of their research. And they have described in some detail how much more we need to know about these important areas of inquiry.

We all look forward to future volumes in the series wherein these and other relevant dimensions of our field will receive the kind and degree of intensive investigative effort exemplified by the contributions to this volume.

BYRON P. ROURKE
UNIVERSITY OF WINDSOR

References

Rourke, B. P., Bakker, D. J., Fisk, J. L., & Strang, J. D. (1983). *Child neuropsychology: An introduction to theory, research, and clinical practice*. New York: Guilford Press.

Preface

The field of child neuropsychology is growing, differentiating, and undergoing dynamic change. Whereas it once occupied a relatively small and often overlooked place within the general field of neuropsychology, it now has become a distinct focus of research and practice. New knowledge is rapidly accumulating, but in many respects the field is still at a rather early formative stage. It is a time when innovative ideas, well-conceptualized questions, and exemplary approaches to complex problems can play an especially critical role in helping to shape future directions and important lines of inquiry.

Advances in Child Neuropsychology is a multi-volume book series that is designed to help highlight, summarize, and critically evaluate important developments in this young but rapidly growing field. It is intended to serve as a forum for exemplary work and critical information spanning a broad range of topics pertinent to researchers and practitioners alike. The topics and contributing authors for each volume are selected with the input of a diversified group of editorial advisors to help assure a balanced representation of major developments and innovations in the field. Collectively, the series should provide a useful and authoritative distillation of information for advanced students and professionals in neuropsychology and related disciplines.

In organizing Volume 1, emphasis was given to soliciting contributions within four general aspects of neuropsychological work and investigation: developmental neuropsychology, abnormal neuropsychology, assessment, and treatment. The goal was to assure a balanced coverage that included topics dealing with therapeutic intervention and normal developmental processes in childhood—areas that too often are overshadowed by an almost exclusive emphasis on assessment and brain damage syndromes. Each chapter was organized to provide either: (1) an authoritative review of a key substantive area or methodological issue in child neuropsychology, or (2) the exposition of an exemplary line of programmatic research or application in the field. In either case, the contribution was to provide an important foundation and possible impetus for future advances in child neuropsychology.

Volume 1 consists of six chapters divided into the four general areas noted above. Part I (developmental neuropsychology) includes a chapter by Dennis L. Molfese that provides an integrated presentation of the findings that have emerged from a series of longitudinal studies on the prediction of language skills using electrophysiological responses recorded from newborn infants. Part II (abnormal neuropsychology) convers a variety of topics dealing with the neurobehavioral effects of selected childhood illnesses or injuries. This includes a chapter on head trauma by Eileen B. Fennell and J. Parker Mickel; one by H. Gerry Taylor, Christopher Schatschneider, and Deborah Rich that investigates the school-age consequences of *Haemophilus influenzae* type b (Hib) meningitis; and a chapter by Alison D. Curley, that examines behavioral disturbance and psychopathology associated with childhood seizures. Of the many possible entries for Part III (assessment), we chose to include a chapter by Kenneth Hugdahl which provides a rigorous but user-friendly overview of dichotic listening procedures with children. Part IV (treatment) focuses on an important and timely topic, cognitive rehabilitation following traumatic head injury, which is discussed through a systematic overview by Mark Ylvisaker, Shirley F. Szekeres, and Patrick Hartwick. Lastly, the volume includes a closing section offering editorial commentary.

We are indebted to a number of individuals for their help at various points in the development of the *Advances* series and the preparation of this volume. Sincere appreciation goes to our distinguished group of editorial advisors for their thoughtful input. In alphabetical order, these include Russell Barkley, Raymond Dean, George Hynd, Francis Pirozzolo, Byron Rourke, Michael Rutter, Paul Satz, Otfried Spreen, and Barbara Wilson. We are also especially grateful to Robert Kidd for his support and helpful guidance at the outset of this project.

MICHAEL G. TRAMONTANA
STEPHEN R. HOOPER

Contents

III. Assessment

IV. Treatment

Contributors

ALISON D. CURLEY
Associates in Mental Health and Neuropsychology
Niandskayuna, New York 12309, USA
and
Consultant to the Hematology Oncology Section
Department of Pediatrics
Albany Medical College
Albany, New York 12208, USA

EILEEN B. FENNELL
Department of Clinical and Health Psychology
University of Florida
Gainesville, Florida 32610, USA

PATRICK HARTWICK
School of Education
State University of New York at Geneseo
Geneseo, New York 14454, USA

KENNETH HUGDAHL
Department of Biological and Medical Psychology
University of Bergen
Bergen, Norway

J. PARKER MICKLE
Department of Neurosurgery
University of Florida
Gainesville, Florida 32610, USA

DENNIS L. MOLFESE
Departments of Psychology and Physiology
Southern Illinois University at Carbondale
Carbondale, Illinois, USA

Deborah Rich
Department of Pediatrics
Case Western Reserve School of Medicine and Rainbow Babies and Childrens Hospital
Cleveland, Ohio 44106, USA

Christopher Schatschneider
Department of Pediatrics
Case Western Reserve University
Cleveland, Ohio 44106, USA

Shirley F. Szekeres
Department of Communication Disorders
Nazareth College of Rochester
Rochester, New York 14618, USA

H. Gerry Taylor
Department of Pediatrics
Case Western Reserve School of Medicine and Rainbow Babies and Childrens Hospital
Cleveland, Ohio 44106, USA

Mark Ylvisaker
Department of Communication Disorders
College of St. Rose
Albany, New York 12203, USA

CHAPTER 1

The Use of Auditory Evoked Responses Recorded from Newborn Infants to Predict Language Skills

DENNIS L. MOLFESE

Over the past two decades, an increasing number of investigations reported that various behavioral and medical measures are useful in characterizing the development of normal infants as well as those infants who may be at risk for a variety of learning disabilities (see V. Molfese, 1989, for a review and evaluation of the effectiveness of these measures). Although such research reports appear promising, the correlations reported and the percentage of variance accounted for are typically low. At best, 50% of the variance has been accounted for in predictive studies utilizing birth measures as predictors of outcomes in the preschool period (Molfese & Molfese, 1985). In an effort to predict more accurately later developmental outcomes, researchers have been turning toward other measures such as the brain stem evoked response and the long latency evoked potential response that might converge with these traditional behavioral assessment measures in order to build better predictive models. Studies utilizing such evoked brain responses have for some time been viewed as providing new information concerning the structural integrity of the brain, insights into brain functioning, and the development of hemispheric involvement in cognitive and language abilities (Callaway, Tueting, & Koslow, 1978).

Along with the use of these more physiologically based measures has come an increased interest in biologically related influences on language acquisition. This is evidenced by the number of journal articles and books dealing with this topic that have recently appeared (see Molfese & Segalowitz, 1988, for reviews of this literature). Lenneberg (1967), for one, argued that a biological substrate exists which subserves language abilities at a number of levels in humans. He clearly linked language acquisition to brain organization. In fact, for him, lateralization of brain functions was a biological sign of language ability (Lenneberg, 1967, p. 67). Although more recent studies have challenged some of Lenneberg's specific hypotheses on lateralization and language development (Dennis & Whitaker, 1977; Molfese, 1972; Molfese, Freeman, & Palermo, 1975), his general view that specific biological underpinnings for language facilitate language development continues to be supported (Dennis & Whitaker, 1977; Molfese & Molfese, 1979a; Molfese & Molfese, 1979b; Molfese & Molfese, 1980; Segalowitz & Gruber, 1977; Molfese & Segalowitz, 1988). The remainder of this chapter addresses two electrophysiological measures which have been used to investigate more thoroughly this relationship, the brainstem auditory evoked response and the event-related potential.

Electrophysiological Measures and Long-Term Prediction

Two regions of the brain's evoked electrical response have been used to study developmental outcomes in young infants: the brainstem evoked response (BSER) and the evoked potential (EP), or event-related potential (ERP). Although both of these responses can be elicited by visual, auditory, or somatosensory stimuli, they differ on a number of dimensions. The BSER generally consists of seven peaks that occur during the first 10–15 ms (milliseconds) of the brain's response. Each peak lasts for a very brief period of time (approximately 1 ms) and the maximum amplitude of this BSER is approximately $\frac{1}{2}$ μV (microvolt). The ERP, on the other hand, is larger in amplitude (range = 5 to 20 μV), slower in frequency, and consists of peaks that are longer in duration than those that characterize the BSER. Whereas the BSER usually is recorded with settings to accept frequencies between 150 and 2000 Hz, the lower frequencies between .1 Hz and 30 to 100 Hz are used to study ERP activity.

Auditory Brainstem Evoked Responses

Beginning in the late 1960s, the BSER technique came to be used more frequently as an objective means for assessing auditory functioning. Usually a very brief visual (i.e., a 1 ms light flash) or auditory (i.e., a 1 ms click) stimulus is used to elicit a BSER. Once elicited, this response is recorded over a 10 to 15 ms period following stimulus onset via "active" electrodes placed at vertex (Cz) and a reference placed at a mastoid (M) site. Although Wave I, Wave III, and Wave V are reliably identified in newborn infants, it is the threshold, amplitude, and latency of Wave V compared to Wave I that has been used most frequently to evaluate auditory functioning (Murray, 1988a, 1988b).

Because exposure to certain perinatal risk events has been associated with hearing loss, several researchers have examined the relationship between perinatal events and abnormalities in BSERs (Barden & Peltzman, 1980; Cox, Hack, & Metz, 1984; Murray, 1988a, 1988b). Barden and Peltzman used the BSER technique with newborn infants, 12 of whom had no risk factors and 15 infants with three or more risk factors. No significant differences between perinatal risk groups in the latency of Wave V were found. Attempts to find group differences in Wave V latencies using birth weight or Apgar scores as the basis for groupings also did not produce significant results. In a later study, Cox, Hack, and Metz studied a population of 50 very low birth weight infants. BSERs were obtained at birth and again at 4 months of age for each infant. Responses were categorized as normal or abnormal (e.g., no response at 60 dB hearing level (HL) or Wave V latency longer than 2 standard devidtions (SD) using normative data from a group of "low-risk preterm infants"; see Cox, Hack, & Metz, 1981). Perinatal risk scores were used in a discriminant function analysis to predict group membership. The perinatal risk scores predicted group membership at birth and at 4 months of age with an accuracy rate of 92% for both time periods. However, of the nine infants with abnormal BSERs at birth, only one was still abnormal at 4 months. In addition, the only other infant who was abnormal at 4 months had not been identified as abnormal at birth.

Murray (1988b) studied 60 high-risk neonates. In this study, instead of relying only on Wave V latency, the latency difference between Waves I and V was used as a measure of BSER abnormality. Less optimal Wave I–Wave V latency differences were found to be associated with specific perinatal risk events [e.g., C-section, use of general anesthesia, low gestational age, low scores on the Obstetrical Complication Scale (Littman & Parmelee, 1978), and postnatal stay in a neonatal intensive care unit]. However, even here, perinatal risk events accounted for only 19% of the variance in regression models to predict Wave I–Wave V latency differences. In a later study, Murray (1988) studied 65 high-risk and 28 low-risk infants on whom data had been obtained at birth and at age 9 months. Using a signal detection approach, the screening sensitivity of the BSERs obtained at birth was evaluated against functioning at later ages. Of the 7 infants with sensorineural hearing loss at 9 months, 5 had been so diagnosed at birth. Six other infants were identified incorrectly at birth as impaired. Of the 3 infants identified as having neuromaturational delay at birth, 2 were confirmed at 9 months. When newborn BSER abnormalities were used to predict the presence of varying levels of neurobehavioral handicaps at 9 months, the accuracy rate was 58% (7 of 12 correctly identified). Interestingly, none of the measures of behavioral audiometry at 9 months differentiated between the newborn BSER groupings.

Although investigators continue their work using BSER to identify possible relationships between the BSER and later developmental outcomes, it is clear, given the findings reviewed here and in Table 1.1, that the procedure has not been effective in identifying infants or children at risk for later developmental problems based on only BSER activity recorded at birth. The number of false positives (i.e., the number of infants identified as at risk for later problems who do not develop such problems) and false negatives (i.e., the number of children who are not

Table 1.1. Attempts to utilize brainstem evoked responses (BSER) recorded from newborn infants to predict cognitive outcomes later in development.

Study	Subjects	Measure	Results
Barden and Peltzman (1980)	15 risk infants 12 no risk infants	BSER—wave V latency	No difference between groups in latency for: Perinatal risk Birth weight Apgar scores
Cox, Hack, and Metz (1984)	50 low birth weight infants tested at birth and at 4 months of age	BSER—wave V latency at 60 dB	Only 11% of infants (i.e., 1 of 9) with abnormal BSER at birth were still abnormal 4 months later
Murray (1988b)	120 neonates: 60 high risk 60 low risk	BSER—latency between wave i and wave V	Perinatal risk accounted for 19% of the variance in predicting latencies
Murray (1988a)	Infants tested at birth and again 9 months later: 65 high risk 28 low risk	BSER—latency between wave i and wave V	5 of 7 infants with sensorineural loss at 9 months were identified at birth 6 infants were incorrectly identified at birth as impaired 2 of 3 newborn infants identified as having neuromaturational delays were confirmed at 9 months of age 58% accuracy in predicting neurobehavioral handicaps at 9 months of age from newborn BSER

identified at birth as at risk for developmental problems but who display some later developmental problems) using this procedure seems much too great to permit the use of the BSER as an effective and efficient screening tool. In addition, only relatively narrow age ranges have been studied to date. To be more efficient, such studies must be conducted that follow infants beyond the first 6 months of life into at least the second, third, and fourth years so that other more complex measures of language and cognitive functioning can be used as end points for the BSER predictive models.

Event-Related Potentials

The ERP has an extensive history as a tool to study language and cognitive processes (see Molfese, 1983, for a review). It is a synchronized portion of the ongoing EEG pattern that is detectable at the scalp and occurs immediately in response to some auditory stimulus (Callaway et al., 1978; Rockstroh, Elbert, Birbaumer, & Lutzenberger, 1982). The ERP is believed to reflect changes in brain activity over time as reflected by changes in the amplitude or height of the waveform at different points in its time course. The ongoing EEG activity reflects a wide range of neural activity related to a variety of body systems, as well as the various sensory and cognitive functions ongoing in the brain at that time. Because of its time-locked relation to the evoking stimulus, the ERP has been demonstrated to reflect both general and specific aspects of the evoking stimulus and the infant's perceptions and decisions regarding it (Molfese, 1983; Molfese & Betz, 1988; Molfese & Molfese, 1979a, 1979b, 1980, 1985; Nelson & Salapatek, 1986; Ruchkin, Sutton, Munson, & Macar, 1981). It is this time-locking feature that enables researchers to identify portions of the brain's electrical response that occur while the infant's attention is focused on some discrete event.

The ERP is not a completely stable electrical pattern that reflects only discrete neural events directly related to the evoking stimulus, the task, or the subject's state. Rather, it is a by-product of the brain's bioelectrical response to such an event, which begins at levels well below that of the cortex as the stimulus information is transformed by the sensory systems. This response progresses through the brainstem, into the midbrain, and upward into the higher centers of the brain. Such signals that originate within the brain must travel through a variety of tissues of different densities, conductivity, and composition (e.g., neurons, glial cells, fiber tracts, cerebrospinal fluid, bone, muscle) before they reach the recording electrodes placed on the scalp. Consequently, the final version of the ERP recorded at the scalp is a composite of a variety of complex factors, only some of which may relate directly to the stimulus situation. Moreover, as changes occur moment-by-moment in these factors, changes will occur at the same time in the amplitude of the ERP waveform which reflect nontask as well as task-related cognitive factors. In addition, the waveshape of the ERP can be changed by the amplifying equipment that is usually set to filter out some or all frequencies above a certain point. Finally, the digitizing process that is used to move these brain responses into our computers can also modify the signal in substantial ways (Goff, 1972; Regan, 1989). Thus there are many factors that may work together or separately to influence the waveshapes of the ERPs that are examined eventually by the investigator.

One advantage of the ERP procedure is that the researcher can employ identical procedures with all participants, regardless of age or species. This greatly enhances the researcher's ability to make direct comparisons between various subject groups to assess comparability of abilities that range from discrimination to complex ideation. Although the waveshapes of the ERPs change from infancy to adulthood, one can assess whether the brain responses recorded from these different populations reliably discriminate between different stimuli, subject groups, and task characteristics. Moreover, the ERP procedures can be used to obtain response information from subjects who cannot or will not respond because of social, language, or maturity factors. Young infants and children certainly fall within this grouping. The ERPs can also provide information concerning both between-hemisphere differences and within-hemisphere differences. Finally, the procedure elicits time-related data that may provide information about the different points in time when such information is detected and processed.

Evoked Potential Studies Using Latency Changes to Predict Later Development

Over the past two decades there have been a number of attempts to predict later development based on EP measures taken within the first week of life (Butler & Engel, 1969; Engel & Fay, 1972; Henderson & Engel, 1974; Jensen & Engel, 1971; Molfese, 1989; Molfese & Molfese, 1985; Molfese & Searock, 1986). As indicated in Table 1.2, these studies have varied in their effectiveness. In general, studies which restricted analyses to a single early peak latency (i.e., usually the first large negative peak, the N1 component), although achieving some success in short-term prediction, have failed to find a long-term relationship between ERPs and later development. Other studies, however, that have examined additional portions of the waveform indicate that ERPs may have some long-term predictive value in assessing later language skills.

Ertl and Schafer (1969) reported significant although somewhat small correlations between visual evoked potential latencies recorded from older children and a variety of IQ tests. In their report, 573 schoolchildren in grades 2, 3, 4, 5, 7, and 8 were tested using the Wechsler Intelligence Scale for Children (WISC), the Primary Mental Abilities Test (PMA), and the Otis Quick-scoring Mental Ability test. In addition, visual evoked responses were recorded from a bipolar electrode placement in front of and behind the C4 electrode site (approximately halfway between the external auditory meatus and the central point at the top of the head; see Jasper, 1958) to 400 photic light flashes, each 1 ms in

Table 1.2. Attempts to utilize event-related potentials recorded from newborn infants to predict language and cognitive performance skills later in development.

Study	Subjects	Measure	Results
Butler and Engel (1969)	433 neonates tested again at 8 months of age	6 channels of EEG/VERP recorded from each hemisphere to light flashes Measured latency to N1 (225 ms) Correlated VER latencies, birth weight, gestational age, and 8 month old performance on Bayley MA, Gross Motor, and Fine Motor scales	Even eliminating infants <2500 gr from study resulted in significant ($p <$ .01) correlations between N1 latency and MA (.31), Fine Motor (.19), and Gross Motor (.20) scales Gestational age also correlated significantly ($p <$ .01) with these at .25, 18, and 16, respectively
Jensen and Engel (1971)	1058 neonates tested again at 1 year	Assessed relation between photic latencies, conceptional age, and percentage of infants walking at 1 year Photic latencies divided into 3 ranges: <146 ms; 146–165 ms; >166 ms	For different conceptional ages, the proportion of infants walking by 1 year of age was greater if the infants had shorter latency responses to photic stimuli as neonates
Engel and Fay (1972)	828 neonates tested again at 3 and 4 years	VER latency measured at P2 from inion referred separately to C3 and C4 Measured speech production of one-syllable words imitated by the child Measured 14 items of comprehension and 5 items of vocal identification of objects	For articulation of initial consonants, fast latency group (<146 ms) performed better than slow reactors (>175 ms) No relationship between neonatal latency and naming or comprehension at 3 years No relationship between VER latency and Stanford-Binet at 4 years

continued

Table 1.2. *Continued*

Study	Subjects	Measure	Results
Henderson and Engel (1974)	809 neonates tested at 1 week and at 7 years of age	VER from Oz referred separately to O_1 and O_2 or from O_1 and O_2 referred separately to C_3 and C_4	No relationship found between neonatal VER amplitudes for N1–P2 and WISC subtest scores
		Measured 7 subtests of WISC at 7 years	
Molfese and Molfese (1985)	16 neonates retested at 3 years of age	At birth, ERPs to speech and nonspeech consonant–vowel sounds recorded from left (T3) and right (T4) temporal areas (Ref = linked ears)	The positive peak of the neonatal Ts response between 88 ms and 240 ms discriminated between consonant sounds for above-average language users at 3 years
		McCarthy test administered at 3 years of age	Positive peak of neonatal response that discriminated consonant–vowel sounds across both hemispheres at 664 ms also characterized only above-average language users at 3 years
Molfese and Searock (1986)	16 one-year-old infants retested at 3 years	At 1 year of age, ERPs recorded to speech and nonspeech vowel sounds from left (T3) and right (T4) hemisphere temporal areas (Ref = linked ears)	Children with above-average language skills at 3 years generated ERPs at 1 year old that discriminated between different vowel sounds
		McCarthy test administered at 3 years of age	
Molfese (1989)	30 neonates retested at 3 years: 15 with McCarthy scores below 50 15 with McCarthy scores above 50	At birth, ERPs to speech and nonspeech consonant–vowel sounds recorded from left (T3) and right (T4) temporal areas (Ref = linked ears) McCarthy test administered at 3 years of age	Discriminant function correctly classified 68.6% of the ERPs recorded from children with McCarthy scores above 50 and 69.7% of the ERPs recorded from children with McCarthy scores below 50

Table 1.2. *Continued*

Study	Subjects	Measure	Results
Molfese (present study)	54 neonates retested at 3 years of age: 27 with McCarthy scores below 50 27 with McCarthy scores above 54	At birth, ERPs recorded to speech and nonspeech consonant–vowel sounds from left and right hemisphere frontal, temporal, and parietal sites (Ref = linked ears)	Positive peak of neonatal left hemisphere responses between 70 ms and 240 ms discriminated between consonant sounds for above-average language users at 3 years
		McCarthy test administered at 3 years of age	Positive peak of neonatal parietal response that discriminated consonant sounds across both hemispheres between 470 and 670 ms also characterized only above-average language users at 3 years

Key: ERP, event-related potential; MA, mental Age subtest; VER, visual evoked response; VERP, visual evoked response potential; WISC, Wechsler Intelligence Scale for Children.

duration. The evoked potentials were filtered such that only frequencies between 3 and 50 Hz were amplified and averaged over 400 presentations for a 625 ms interval from stimulus onset. Using both a zero-crossing analysis and an amplitude summation procedure to cross-validate peak identifications, Ertl and Schafer measured the stimulus onset to peak latencies for four negative peaks from 32.8 to 187.4 ms. In general, they found that IQ scores correlated best with later peak latencies, although the range of the correlations continued to be small. For example, WISC Full Scale IQ correlated −.18, −.30, −.35, and −.33 with peaks 1, 2, 3, and 4, respectively. Ertl and Schafer concluded from these findings that "evoked potentials which reflect the time course of information processing by the brain, could be the key to understanding the biological substrate of individual differences in behavioral intelligence" (p. 422).

Butler and Engel (1969) reported the first success in this area in testing brain responses from young infants and noting some correlations between the neonatal evoked potential latencies and later measures related to intelligence. They recorded visual evoked potentials during the first 5 days of life from 433 newborn infants in response to a series of photic flashes. The mothers of the infants were part of a random sample from a clinic serving a low socioeconomic status (SES) metropolitan population on the West Coast of the United States. Like Ertl (1969), Butler and Engel chose to measure peak latencies to a negative component and recorded the photic response latency for what they labeled as N1. This period extended from stimulus onset until the initial large negative peak that occurred approximately 225 ms later. Henderson and Engel noted that this latency could be identified as the "interval between stimulus onset and the takeoff point (N1) that leads to the peak P2" (Henderson & Engel, 1974, p. 271). Subsequent behavioral tests were made of each infant's Mental (e.g., responses to objects, vocalizations), Gross Motor (e.g., sitting, stepping, pulling up), and Fine Motor (hand and finger dexterity, etc.) behaviors at 8 months of age using the Bayley Scales of Children's Abilities. Correlations were then computed between the neonatal photic latency, gestational age, duration of pregnancy, birth weight, and these Mental, Gross Motor, and Fine Motor skills. Although the correlations were significant between the motor behaviors and photic latency, the effects were small and accounted for little of the variance. Photic latency significantly correlated with Mental ($r = .33$, $p < .01$), Fine Motor ($r = .24$, $p < .01$), and Gross Motor ($r = .23$, $p < .01$) behaviors. It is interesting to note that comparable significant correlations were found between the Bayley measures and gestational age ($r = .31$, .26, .23, respectively; all effects were beyond $p < .001$), whereas somewhat less notable correlations were found for birth weight ($r = .18$, .15, .12, respectively; the effects ranged from $p < .001$ to $p < .01$ to $p < .05$, respectively).

Jensen and Engel (1971) also reported correlations between neonatal photic latencies and later motor skills. In this case, they divided the photic latency response centered around the N1 peak identified by Butler and Engel (1969) into three regions and correlated these three latency regions with whether the infant was walking at the time of a 1 year follow-up exam that occurred at approximately 1 year of age. Infants were divided into those whose N1 latency was less than 146 ms, those whose latency ranged between 146 and 165 ms, and those infants with N1 latencies beyond 166 ms. These data then were plotted for conceptional age, and a percentage walking in each category was determined. Separate linear functions then were derived for each group and these functions were tested against a single regression function for the entire sample of infants. The test indicated that indeed separate functions appeared to describe each of the three latency groups. Thus, in general, Jensen and Engel found that "the proportion of walking tends to be greater, the shorter the adjusted latency of response to photic stimulus in the neonate" (p. 441).

In a subsequent study, Engel and Fay (1972) also measured the visual evoked response N1 latency and tested for possible relationships between this latency and early articulation of initial consonant sounds, naming, comprehension at 3 years of age, and Stanford-Binet IQ at 4 years of age.

The final sample included 828 infants. As in the Butler and Engel (1969) and Jensen and Engel (1971) studies, the children were drawn from a low SES population. The 3 year language tests consisted of 14 items of the standard comprehension subtest plus 5 vocal identifications of familiar objects in real or toy form. The children's responses during the comprehension test were nonvocal and consisted of the manual identification and manipulation of familiar objects in response to the tester's requests. The speech test included articulation of one-syllable words that were initially produced by a speech pathologist and repeated by the child. Articulation measures then were based upon 23 initial consonants and 21 final consonants contained within these words. Following testing, the children were assigned to one of two language groups (high vs. low) by means of a median split based upon these measures. Next, the children were divided into three groups based upon their visual evoked response (VER) N1 latencies in order to determine whether a relationship existed between their brain wave latency and language skills. These groups, however, differed from those proposed and used earlier by Jensen and Engel. Instead, Engel and Fay constructed a "fast latency" group based on latencies less than 146 ms and a "slow reactors" group with latencies longer than 175ms.

Results indicated that for initial and final consonant articulation, the fast-reactor group (latencies less than 146 ms) performed better at 3 years of age than the slow reactors. Overall, females were better than males. A subsequent analysis of photic latencies for 1046 children at 4 years of age showed a significant effect only for the black females ($p < .05$) but no other effects. The authors hypothesized that this finding was a chance effect and dismissed it from further consideration, concluding that "photic latency measurements of term infants do not appear to be valid predictors of the Stanford-Binet at four-years-of-age" (p. 286).

Subsequent studies with older populations of children conducted by Engel and Henderson (1973) and Henderson and Engel (1974) also failed to find any relationship between neonatal visual evoked responses and a variety of later IQ and achievement scores. Engel and Henderson, in analyzing visual evoked response latencies recorded from the left inion site[1] over the back of the head from a group of 119 children between 7 and 8 years of age, found no relationship between various latency measures of the waveform for each child and the child's performance

[1] It is difficult in reading the Engel and Henderson (1973) paper to determine exactly what sites were used for the latency measures. On page 136 reference is made to recording from 15 electrode sites. However, in column 2 of page 137 latency measures are given for the positive and negative peaks over the inion site. Additionally, whereas they note that electrode references were placed over the left and right sides, they state that "measurements were taken from the left tracing" (p. 137).

on a number of subtests of the WISC that included Information, Comprehension, Vocabulary, and Digit Span as well as the Picture Arrangement, Block Design, and Coding subtests. Additionally, they tested relationships between these brain wave measures and the scores obtained from the Bender-Gestalt Test. In a subsequent paper, Henderson and Engel (1974) speculated that the possible relationships previously reported between evoked potential latencies and later intelligence could have resulted from a number of problems. These included the reliability of the visual evoked response latencies and amplitudes of the waveforms in young infants, the attention given to a relatively small number of significant correlations while the much greater number of nonsignificant effects were ignored, and the tendency of some researchers to compare neurologically normal with neurologically abnormal populations. In the latter case, abnormal EEG tracings could have contributed significantly to the success in predicting later development if for no other reason than children who might be characterized early by grossly abnormal EEG patterns would have serious resulting cognitive disabilities that would make them less likely to develop normal cognitive skills. One point, however, that Engel and Henderson (1973) failed to note was that different electrode sites were used in their study than in those employed by earlier investigators. Such differences could have contributed to the lack of agreement between the findings of their study and the earlier work conducted by Ertl (1971).

In a further attempt to determine whether some relationship might exist between early brain responses and later IQ in normal children, Henderson and Engel (1974) assessed whether the neonatal visual evoked responses of children would predict their total IQ and subtest scores, sensorimotor, perceptual-motor, and achievement test scores at 7 years of age. In this study, they drew a sample of 809 neonates from the same population as the other studies involving Engel and his collaborators. The photic latency data from these infants then were correlated with their performance on a variety of WISC subtests (Information, Comprehension, Vocabulary, Digit Span, Picture Arrangement, Block Design, and Coding) as well as the WISC Full Scale, Verbal, and Performance IQ scores, the Bender-Gestalt Test, the Tactile Finger Recognition Test (adapted from the Reitan-Indiana Neuropsychological Battery for Children), and the spelling, reading, and arithmetic tests from the Wide Range Achievement Test. These tests were administered to the children between 6 years, 10 months and 7 years, 3 months of age.

After correcting the neonatal latency data for prematurity and discarding subjects from the sample who had not completed all of the behavioral tests or whose Full Scale IQ scores were 2.5 standard deviations below their cohort in this study, the scores were stepwise regressed on the visual evoked response and calculations determined both partial regression coefficients and multiple correlations. Regressions were conducted separately for each race (i.e., blacks and whites) and sex. None of the regression coefficients of neonatal visual evoked responses on IQs were significant. Whereas some of the scores were in the expected direction, none of the simple or multiple correlations of the evoked potential latency with the outcome variables differed from chance levels. The authors concluded that, at least for "neurologically normal children, neonatal photic latency is not related to IQ seven years later; nor is it related to subtests that contribute to IQ, achievement, or to perceptual-motor and sensory-perceptual responses" (Henderson & Engel, 1974, p. 275).

From the preceding review, it appears that several studies do suggest some early relationship between one component of the visual evoked response, the latency or length of the interval between stimulus onset and the N1 peak, and subsequent motor, cognitive-motor, or language-related abilities up to 3 years of age (Butler & Engel, 1969; Engel & Fay, 1972; Henderson & Engel, 1974; Jensen & Engel, 1971). However, further research which compared early neonatal evoked responses with later intelligence score measures failed to demonstrate a relationship between these evoked potential measures and subsequent IQ development beyond 3 years. Although such conclusions may appear discouraging, more recent studies from a number of laboratories suggest that relationships might in fact exist between early evoked responses and later measures of intelligence (Molfese, 1989; Molfese & Molfese, 1985; Molfese & Searock, 1986).

However, if so many previous studies failed to find reliable and robust relationships between neonatal evoked potentials and later intelligence measures, how could other studies identify such relationships? Would not this inconsistency across studies suggest that the evoked potential methodology itself is subject to problems of reliability and stability? In fact, the differences among such studies and their success or failure to find such relationships may reflect a number of differences in both methodology and experimental design. The studies reported by Molfese and his associates differ from those of Ertl and others in that the entire evoked potential waveform is subjected to data analysis instead of a single peak. Such a strategy might increase the likelihood of finding a relationship between early brain responses and later development, if such relationships do in fact exist. Moreover, the frequency range of the evoked potential studied in these subjects includes a lower range of frequencies than those employed by the other investigators discussed here. Given that the brain wave frequencies that characterize the evoked potentials of young infants are concentrated in the frequency range below 3 Hz, such a strategy should increase the likelihood of obtaining more of the neonate's brain wave activity. Finally, these later studies employ stimuli that are clearly language-related speech sounds. Perhaps the inclusion of more language-relevant stimuli might increase the likelihood of improving the prediction of later language-related skills.

Evoked Potential Studies Using Amplitude Changes to Predict Later Development

Molfese and Molfese, in addition to investigating changes in developmental patterns of lateralization across the life span, have isolated and identified electrophysiological correlates of various speech perception cues across and within a number of developmental periods (Molfese, 1989; Molfese & Molfese, 1979a, 1985). One major issue recently raised concerns the implications of these lateralized patterns of response for later language development. Are these patterns of responses related to later language development for individual children or do they reflect some basic pattern of auditory processing in the brain that has little relation to language development? Given Lenneberg's (1967) notion that lateralization is a biological sign of language, could such early patterns of lateralized discrimination of speech sounds predict later language outcomes? Theoreticians have speculated that the absence of hemispheric differences in a child indicates that the child is at risk for certain cognitive or language disabilities (Travis, 1931). Although the data generally have not supported such a position, it is possible that predictions concerning later performance could be enhanced when hemispheric differences are considered in light of specific processing capacities.

In this regard, Molfese and Molfese (1985, 1986) attempted to establish the validity of a variety of factors in predicting long-term outcomes in language development from measures taken shortly after birth and during the first years of life. Measures used included demographic variables, behavioral scales, and ERPs. The specific issue under study concerned whether general hemispheric differences per se or specific lateralized discrimination abilities would do better in identifying children who later would develop poorer language skills.

In the first study, 16 infants were studied longitudinally from birth through their 3 year birthday. During this time information was collected on factors such as gender, birth weight, length, gestational age, scores on the Obstetric Complications Scale (Littman & Parmelee, 1978), the Brazelton Neonatal Assessment Scale (Als, Tronick, Lester, & Brazelton, 1977; Brazelton, 1973), the Bayley Scales of Infant Development (Bayley, 1969), the Peabody Picture Vocabulary Test (Dunn, 1965), and the McCarthy Scales of Children's Abilities (McCarthy, 1972). Parental ages, incomes, educational levels, and occupations also were obtained. In addition, ERPs were recorded from the left and right temporal areas (T3 and T4) at birth and again at 6 month intervals through the child's third birthday in response to the synthetic speech stimuli employed by Molfese (1980) and Molfese and Schmidt (1983). These stimuli were chosen because they had been found to produce reliable general hemispheric difference effects as well as bilateral and lateralized discrimination effects. In addition, eight other stimulus tokens were added to the auditory ERP test battery in order to facilitate tests of generalizability across the different consonant and vowel contrasts. Such stimuli appeared to be ideally suited for determining whether general hemispheric differences per se or specific lateralized discrimination abilities were the best predictors of later language skills.

Analyses of the auditory ERP data did in fact indicate that electrophysiological measures recorded at birth could identify children who performed better or worse on language tasks 3 years later. Moreover, the best predictor of later language development was the presence of a lateralized speech sound discrimination ability. The newborn infants in whom left-hemisphere–generated ERPs reliably discriminated between the different consonant sounds at birth were more likely to develop better language skills 3 years later. Children who performed poorer at 3 years of age failed to make such discriminations as newborn infants.

Evoked potential activity recorded from the temporal electrode sites under certain stimulus conditions discriminated between the two groups of children. One component of the auditory ERP that occurred between 88 and 240 ms reliably discriminated between children whose index scores were above 50 (the High group) on the McCarthy Scales of Children's Abilities and those who scored lower (i.e., the Low group). Only the ERPs recorded from over the left hemisphere of the High group systematically discriminated between the different consonant speech sounds. The right-hemisphere responses of this group, on the other hand, discriminated between the different nonspeech stimuli. However, the Low group displayed no such lateralized discrimination for either the speech or the nonspeech sounds. A second portion of the auditory ERP with a late peak latency of 664 ms also discriminated between the High and Low groups. Unlike the earlier peak, however, this component occurred over both hemispheres and, consequently, reflected bilateral activity. This second component did not behave in exactly the same manner as the first. It was able to discriminate between speech and nonspeech stimuli. In addition, its ability to discriminate between consonant sounds depended on which vowel followed the consonant. In other words, this auditory ERP component was much more context sensitive. A third segment of the auditory ERP (peak latency = 450 ms) that varied only across hemispheres failed to discriminate between the two different groups. Thus it appears that hemispheric differences per se were not sufficient to discriminate at birth between infants who would develop better or poorer language skills 3 years later. Furthermore, given that the auditory ERP components that discriminated between the two groups were sensitive to certain speech and nonspeech contrasts but not to others, it appears that the ERPs reflected the infant's sensitivity to specific language-related cues rather than the overall readiness of the brain to respond to any general stimulus in its environment.

A stepwise multiple regression model of these data was developed using the Peabody and McCarthy Verbal Index scores as the dependent variables and the ERP components obtained at birth that best discriminated the different consonant sounds as the independent variables. This model accounted for 78% of the total variance in predicting McCarthy scores from the brain responses, whereas 69% of the variance was accounted for in predicting Peabody scores (Molfese & Molfese, 1986). Clearly, there appears to be a strong relationship between early ERP discrimination of speech-related stimuli and later language skills.

A subsequent study by Molfese and Searock (1986) noted that this relationship between early ERP activity and later language skills continues to exist at 1 year of age. ERPs were recorded from 16 infants within 2 weeks of their first birthday. A series of three vowel sounds with speech formant structure and three nonspeech tokens containing formants 1 Hz wide that matched the mean frequencies of the speech sounds were presented to these infants, and their auditory ERPs were recorded in response to each sound. Two regions of the ERPs, one centered between 300 and 400 ms and another centered around 200 ms following stimulus onset, discriminated between the 1-year-old infants who 2 years later would perform better or worse on the McCarthy language tasks. Infants who were able to discriminate between more vowel sounds performed better on the language tasks at 3 years of age.

In a subsequent study that expanded upon the procedures employed by Molfese and Molfese (1985), Molfese (1989) recorded the auditory evoked responses at birth from scalp electrodes placed over frontal, temporal (T3 and T4; see Jasper, 1958), and parietal scalp areas over the left and right hemispheres. The left and right frontal sites were positioned halfway between Fz and the auditory meatus for the left and right sides of the head. Likewise, the parietal electrodes were positioned halfway between Pz and the auditory meatus for the left and right sides of the head. These active recording sites were referred to linked ear references. As in the case of Molfese and Molfese (1985), the testing was carried out on the infants within 24 hours of birth. The speech and nonspeech sounds that served as stimuli were a subset of those employed by Molfese and Molfese (1985) and consisted of the speech syllables [bi, gi] and the nonspeech analogues for these two consonant–vowel sounds. These four sounds had been found to be the best predictors from the earlier study.

After the electrodes were attached to the infant's scalp, the infant's bed was positioned at 40 degrees from horizontal beneath a speaker such that the speaker was 1 meter above the center of the infant's head and equidistant from each ear. Ongoing EEG activity was monitored throughout the testing. Stimulus presentation began once the EEG patterns indicated that the infant was in a quiet awake state. Stimulus presentation and data collection were interrupted periodically in some infants when the infants became more active. Testing then would recommence upon cessation of movement. The auditory evoked responses were amplified at 20,000 and recorded onto FM cassette tape using a Vetter C8 FM system along with two pulses, one a 20 μV calibration pulse and the other a trigger pulse that identified the onset of an auditory stimulus so that a computer later could identify the beginning of a trial for data collection. Following testing the ERPs from each electrode site and for each stimulus were screened separately for artifacts and then averaged using a Macintosh microcomputer system and the EPACS software package for evoked potential analysis. These averaged ERPs were used as the basis for the discriminant function procedures described later.

Additional data on perinatal risk conditions were obtained from medical records and demographic information was obtained from the parents. The infants were brought back at their first, second, and third birthday for behavioral retesting, additional ERP testing, and to update demographic and health history information on each infant. The behavioral tests at 1 year of age were from the Bayley Scales of Infant Development, at 2 years of age the Bayley Scales and the revised Stanford-Binet Intelligence Scale (Thorndike, Hagen, & Sattler, 1986), and at 3 years of age the revised Stanford-Binet, the McCarthy Scales of Children's Abilities (McCarthy, 1972), and the Peabody Picture Vocabulary Test–Revised. In addition, at 3 years of age a home visit was made to obtain information on the HOME Scale (Caldwell & Bradley, 1978) and to complete the behavioral testing. This sample of 30 infants had McCarthy verbal scores at 3 years of age that ranged from 32 to 69 (M = 53, sd = 9.41). The mean for the infants who scored 50 or below on the McCarthy test was 45 (sd = 4.97, range = 32–50). The mean for the infants who scored above 50 was 61 (sd = 4.95, range = 54–69). These children, then, comprised a sample of subjects who possessed largely average language scores. Data from both risk and nonrisk infants were collected during this study, but the data set reported by Molfese concerned only a group of normal infants. As was the case with Engel and his associates, Molfese attempted to determine whether brain responses at birth could be used to discriminate among relatively *normal* infants whose language skills 3 years later would fall *within the normal range*.

A Discriminant Function Procedure was applied to the newborn ERPs. The time points of the averaged ERPs were used to discriminate the language scores obtained when the subjects were 3 years of age. In this analysis the averaged ERPs were divided into two groups, those obtained from infants who 3 years later scored above 50 on the McCarthy test and those who scored below 50. The stepwise analysis, with an F-to-enter of 3.0, selected 17 points in order of their effectiveness in classifying each of the 720 original averaged ERPs into one of the two groups. As Molfese noted, these points clustered in four regions of the ERP, the first between 20 and 140 ms, the second between 230 and 270 ms, the third between 410 and 490 ms, and the fourth between 600 and 700 ms. In this analysis, the likelihood of correctly classifying a brain response as belonging to a Low or High language performance child was 50%. The actual classification accuracy, however, was significantly higher than chance. For the

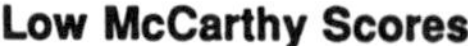

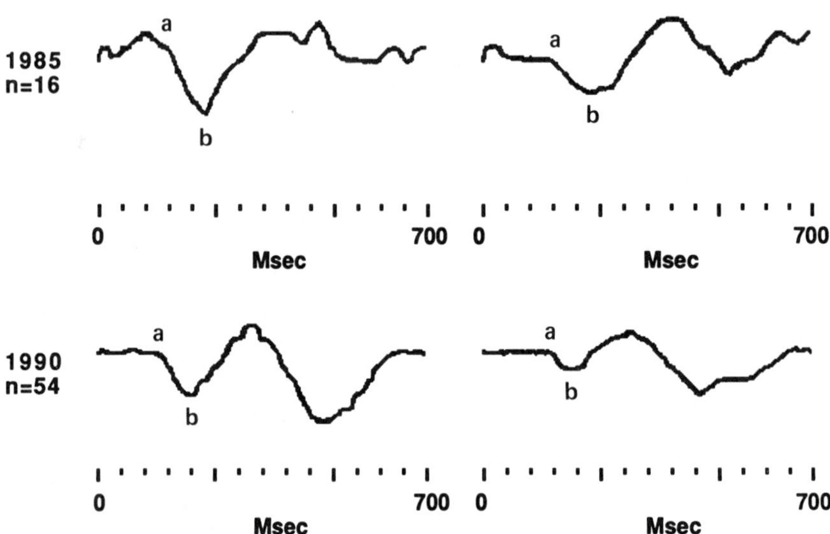

Fig. 1.1. Event-related potential differences recorded from two separate populations of newborn infants, as reported by Molfese and Molfese (1985) and in the present chapter, that predict later language performance skills in these children at 3 years of age.

children who scored above 50 on the McCarthy verbal subtest, the classification was accurate 68.6% of the time, whereas it was accurate 69.7% of the time for the children scoring 50 or below. A Z test of proportions indicated that the actual classification was significantly better than chance for each group ($z = 10.57$, $p < .001$, and $z = 9.98$, $p < .001$, respectively).

As illustrated in Figure 1.1, there are a number of regions of the ERP waveforms that distinguish between the brain waves of infants who will later develop differently in language skills. The upper figures are from the data published by Molfese and Molfese (1985). As reported in that study, two major regions of the waves discriminated between groups. The waveform on the left is the averaged ERP for the eight neonates who at 3 years of age obtained a verbal subtest score on the McCarthy of 20.5 (sd = 12.6), whereas that on the right is the average waveform for the eight infants who obtained an average score of 77.25 (sd = 15.5). The first region involved a positive peak and the leading edge of the following negative wave which occurred between 88 and 240 ms. The second region that discriminated between the two groups of infants began with the most negative peak at approximately 550 ms and continued to the end of the waveform.

In Molfese and Molfese (1985), the initial positive peak is larger for the Low than for the High group. This is reflected in the area shaded with blocks above the horizontal baseline marker. The next positive peak region, however, is larger for the High than for the Low group. Finally, the late negative area is larger for the Low than for the High group.

Recently, data have been collected from a second and larger sample of infants. The stimulus set, data collection, and analyses procedures used in the Molfese (1989) study outlined earlier were employed here as well. In this case, a sample of 1296 ERPs were recorded from 54 children at birth. The language performance of these children was measured with the McCarthy Scales of Children's Abilities at 3 years of age. Half of the children scored above 54 (range = 54–72) on the McCarthy test, whereas the other half scored 50 or below (range = 32–50). The data analysis employed was fashioned after that used by Molfese and Molfese (1985). In this case, a median split separated the infants into two distinct groups, a Low group and a High group. Analyses identified seven regions of variability that accounted for approximately 56% of the total variance. Furthermore, three of these regions varied as a function of the groups' 3 year language performance (Low vs. High). As in the case of Molfese and Molfese (1985), one region between 70 and 210 ms with a peak latency of 140 ms discriminated between groups. The left-hemisphere auditory evoked responses from the High language group discriminated between the two consonant sounds, /b/ and /g/, $F(1,52) = 8.37$, $p < .0057$. This was not the case for the Low language group. The waveforms for these two groups of infants are presented at the bottom of Figure 1.1. The newborn averaged ERP for the 27 children whose average McCarthy Verbal Index score at 3 years of age was 50 or below is presented on the lower left of the figure ($M = 45$, $sd = 4.97$), whereas the averaged ERP on the bottom right was produced by 27 children whose average McCarthy score was 54 or above ($M = 61$, $sd = 4.95$). This effect is especially exciting because it is similar in both latency and lateralized effect to the results of the High language performance group reported by Molfese and Molfese (1985), even though a different and more homogeneous population of infants was used and the stimulus set was a small subset of that employed by Molfese and Molfese.

A second portion of the newborn evoked response in the present data set also discriminated between consonant sounds for the High language group but not for the Low group. In this case, the portion of the left- and right-hemisphere parietal waveforms between 480 and 620 ms discriminated between consonant sounds for the High group [$F(1,104) = 27.58$, $p < .00001$] but not for the Low group. Thus far, then, results from a new and larger longitudinal sample continue to support the earlier findings of Molfese and Molfese (1985).

One interpretation of these results is that early discrimination abilities relate directly to later language development. The children who performed better on language tasks at age 3 discriminated between consonant sounds alone (Molfese, 1989; Molfese & Molfese, 1985) and consonant sounds in combination with different vowel sounds (Molfese & Molfese, 1985). Such a pattern of responding suggests that more linguistically advanced children are already at an advantage at birth because their nervous systems can make finer discriminations along a variety of different dimensions. As Molfese suggests, "Perhaps the earlier an infant can discriminate between speech sounds in its environment, the more likely that infant will be able to use such information to discriminate sound differences" (1989, p. 55). Such early discrimination abilities may later play a major role in the young infant's early word learning. Infants who are facile at speech sound discrimination may find the task of learning to discriminate between words with similar speech sounds easier than the child who cannot readily hear the sound differences and who must rely on less obvious acoustic or contextual clues at perhaps a later point in development.

Conclusions

These data provide further support for the position that early physiological indices can be used to predict long-term developmental trends. One aspect of these data that is especially striking concerns the range of the language abilities that are differentiated approximately 4 years after the brain responses were recorded initially from newborn infants. Whereas the language skills of the Molfese and Molfese (1985) study covered a considerable range from relatively poor receptive and productive skills to well above average skills, the language skills in the present study and in Molfese (1989) are from children whose language skills covered a much more narrow range and were generally much more similar. In fact, the range of language measures place these children generally within or close to the normal range of skills found in children of this age. In spite of this degree of similarity, the brain responses continue to distinguish children who perform differently on the language tasks. Consequently, ERPs collected at birth appear to predict with a high degree of accuracy relatively minor differences in language abilities 4 years later.

These findings, if they continue to hold up as more infants are tested and followed into their later preschool and elementary school years, may portend a radically new and highly accurate type of assessment tool. Until now, no tests have succeeded in predicting later developmental outcomes based on newborn infant measures. Perhaps this limitation has resulted from our reliance on measuring the limited behavioral repertoire of the young infant and the basic lack of commonality or extension of these responses to later behaviors more directly related to cognitive and communicative abilities. Perhaps such limitations have resulted from our own lack of clarity in identifying and adequately describing the behavior we associate with such outcome measures. Whatever the case, it now appears that at least some success has been achieved in relating early neonatal measures to later behaviors. The findings of such relationships between later cognitive skills and early neuroelectrical responses, although still tentative, could provide the basis for an early neuroelectrical screening test to identify children at birth or shortly afterward who may be at risk for later language development problems. The success of such an endeavor, obviously, could dramatically enhance our ability to intervene at an earlier point in the developmental period and possibly remediate factors that could otherwise prevent a child from developing normally. Clearly, there is much work yet to do.

Acknowledgments. Supported by grants from the March of Dimes Birth Defects Foundation (12-142) and National Insitutes of Health (R01 HD17860).

References

Als, H., Tronick, E., Lester, B., & Brazelton, T. (1977). The Brazelton Neonatal Behavioral Assessment Scale (BNAS). *Journal of Abnormal Child Psychology*, *5*, 215–231.

Barden, T., & Peltzman, P. (1980). Newborn brain stem auditory evoked responses and perinatal clinical events. *American Journal of Obstetrics and Gynocology*, *136*, 912–919.

Bayley, N. (1969). *Bayley Scales of Infant Development: Birth to Two Years*. New York: Psychological Corporation.

Brazelton, T. B. (1973). *Neonatal Behavioral Assessment Scale* (Clinics in Developmental Medicine No. 50). Philadelphia: Lippincott.

Butler, B. V., & Engel, R. (1969). Mental and motor scores at 8 months in relation to neonatal photic responses. *Developmental Medicine and Child Neurology*, *11*, 77–82.

Caldwell, B., & Bradley, R. (1978). *Manual of the home observation for measurement of environment*. Unpublished manuscript available from the authors. University of Arkansas, Little Rock.

Callaway, E., Tueting, P., & Koslow, S. (1978). *Event-related brain potentials and behavior*. New York: Academic Press.

Corballis, M. (1983). *Human laterality*. New York: Academic Press.

Cox, C., Hack, M., & Metz, D. (1981). Brainstem-evoked response audiometry: Normative data from the preterm infant. *Audiology*, *20*, 53–64.

Cox, L., Hack, M., & Metz, D. (1984). Auditory brain stem response abnormalities in the very low birthweight infant: Incidence and risk factors. *Ear and Hearing*, *5*, 47–51.

Dennis, M., & Whitaker, H. (1977). Hemispheric equipotentiality and language acquisition. In S. Segalowitz & F. Gruber (Eds.), *Language development and neurological theory* (pp. 93–106). New York: Academic Press.

Dunn, L. (1965). *Peabody Picture Vocabulary Test*. Circle Pines, MN: American Guidance Service.

Engel, R., & Fay, W. (1972). Visual evoked responses at birth, verbal scores at three years, and IQ at four years. *Developmental Medicine and Child Neurology*, *14*, 283–289.

Engel, R., & Henderson, N. B. (1973). Visual evoked responses and IQ scores at school age. *Developmental Medicine and Child Neurology*, *15*, 136–145.

Ertl, J. P. (1971). Fourier analysis of evoked potentials and human intelligence. *Nature*, *230*, 525–526.

Ertl, J. P. & Schafer, E. W. P. (1969). Brain response correlates of psychometric intelligence. *Nature*, *223*, 421–422.

Goff, W. R. Human average evoked potentials: procedures for stimulating and recording. In R. F. Thompson & M. M. Patterson, (Eds.), *Bioelectric recording techniques, Part B*. New York: Academic Press, 101–156.

Henderson, N. B., & Engel, R. (1974). Neonatal visual evoked potentials as predictors of psychoeducational testing at age seven. *Developmental Psychology*, *10*, 269–276.

Jasper, H. H. (1958). The ten-twenty electrode system of the International Federation of Societies for Electroencephalography: Appendix to report of the committee on methods of clinical examination in electroencephalography. *Electroencephalography and Clinical Neurophysiology*, *10*, 371–375.

Jensen, D. R., & Engel, R. (1971). Statistical procedures for relating dichotomous responses to maturation and EEG measurements. *Electroencephalography and Clinical Neurophysiology*, *30*, 437–443.

Lenneberg, E. (1967). *Biological foundations of language*. New York: Wiley.

Littman, B., & Parmelee, A. (1978). Medical correlates of infant development. *Pediatrics*, *61*, 470–474.

McCarthy, D. (1972). *Manual for the McCarthy Scales of Children's Abilities*. New York: Psychological Corporation.

Molfese, D. L. (1972). *Cerebral asymmetry in infants, children and adults: Auditory evoked responses to speech and noise stimuli*. Dissertation accepted by the Department of Psychology, The Pennsylvania State University.

Molfese, D. L. (1980). The phoneme and the engram: Electrophysiological evidence for the acoustic invariant in stop consonants. *Brain and Language*, *9*, 372–376.

Molfese, D. L. (1983). Event related potentials and language processes. In A. W. K. Gaillard & W. Ritter (Eds.), *Tutorials in ERP research: Endogenous components* (pp. 345–368). The Hague: North Holland Publishing Co.

Molfese, D. L., & Betz, J. C. (1988). Electrophysiological indices of the early development of lateralization for language and cognition, and their implication for predicting later development. In D. L. Molfese & S. J. Segalowitz (Eds.), *Brain lateralization in children: Developmental implications* (pp. 171–190). New York: Guilford Press.

Molfese, D. L., Freeman, R., & Palermo, D. (1975). The ontogeny of lateralization for speech and nonspeech stimuli. *Brain and Language*, *2*, 356–368.

Molfese, D. L., & Molfese, V. J. (1979a). Hemisphere and stimulus differences as reflected in the cortical responses of newborn infants to speech stimuli. *Developmental Psychology*, *15*, 505–511.

Molfese, D. L., & Molfese, V. J. (1979b). Infant speech perception: Learned or innate? In H. Whitaker & H. Whitaker (Eds.), *Advances in neurolinguistics* (Vol. 4, pp. 225–240). New York: Academic Press.

Molfese, D. L., & Molfese, V. J. (1980). Cortical responses of preterm infants to phonetic and nonphonetic speech stimuli. *Developmental Psychology*, *16*, 574–581.

Molfese, D. L., & Molfese, V. J. (1985). Electrophysiological indices of auditory discrimination in newborn infants: The bases for predicting later language development? *Infant Behavior and Development*, *8*, 197–211.

Molfese, D. L., & Molfese, V. J. (1986). Psychophysical indices of early cognitive processes and their relationship to language. In J. E. Obrzut & G. W. Hynd (Eds.), *Child neuropsychology, Volume 1: Theory and research* (pp. 95–116). New York: Academic Press.

Molfese, D. L., & Molfese, V. J. (1988). Right hemisphere responses from preschool children to temporal cues contained in speech and nonspeech materials: Electrophysiological correlates. *Brain and Language*, *33*, 245–259.

Molfese, D. L., & Schmidt, A. (1983). An auditory evoked potential study of consonant perception in different vowel environments. *Brain and Language*, *18*, 57–70.

Molfese, D. L., & Searock, K. (1986). The use of auditory evoked responses at one year of age to predict language skills at 3 years. *Australian Journal of Communication Disorders*, *14*, 35–46.

Molfese, D. L., & Segalowitz, S. J. (1988). *Brain lateralization in children: Developmental implications*. New York: Guilford Press.

Molfese, V. J. (1989). *Perinatal risk and infant development: Assessment and prediction*. New York: Guilford Press.

Molfese, V. J., & Holcomb, L. C. (1989). Predicting learning and other developmental disabilities: Assessment of reproductive and caretaker variables. In N. W. Paul (Ed.), *Research in infant assessment* (pp. 1–24). New York: March of Dimes Birth Defects Foundation.

Murray, A. (1988). Newborn auditory brainstem evoked responses (ABRs): Longitudinal correlates in the first year. *Child Development*, *59*, 1542–1554.

Murray, A., Dolby, R., Nation, R., & Thomas, D. (1981). Effects of epidural anesthesia on newborns and their mothers. *Child Development*, *52*, 71–82.

Nelson, C. A., & Salapatek, P. (1986). Electrophysiological correlates of infant recognition memory. *Child Development*, *57*, 1482–1497.

Regan, D. (1989). *Human Brain Electrophysiology*. Amsterdam, The Netherlands: Elseviev.

Rockstroh, B., Elbert, T., Birbaumer, N., & Lutzenberger, W. (1982). *Slow brain potentials and behavior*. Baltimore: Urban & Schwarzenberg.

Ruchkin, D., Sutton, S., Munson, R., & Macar, F. (1981). P300 and feedback provided by the absence of the stimulus. *Psychophysiology*, *18*, 271–282.

Segalowitz, S. (1983). *Language functions and brain organization*. New York: Academic Press.

Segalowitz, S., & Gruber, F. (1977). *Language development and neurological theory*. New York: Academic Press.

Thorndike, R. L., Hagen, E. P., & Sattler, J. M. (1986). *Stanford-Binet Intelligence Scale* (4th ed.). Chicago: The Riverside Publishing Co.

Travis, L. E. (1931). *Speech pathology*. New York: Appleton-Century.

Chapter 2

Behavioral Effects of Head Trauma in Children and Adolescents

Eileen B. Fennell and J. Parker Mickle

Traumatic head injury in children poses a significant health problem because it is a leading cause of death or permanent disability in the pediatric age group (Guyer & Ellers, 1990). Fletcher, Miner, and Ewing-Cobbs (1987) recently estimated that for every 30 newborn infants, 1 will have a significant brain injury before he or she obtains a license to drive. Increasing evidence suggests that head trauma causing even minor brain injury can lead to a variety of behavioral changes that may adversely affect the injured child's ability to meet developmental tasks in the home, at school, and with peers. In this chapter, we review the current literature on the epidemiology of head injuries in children, the causes of pediatric head trauma, and the pathophysiology of several types of head trauma. Research on the neuropsychological consequences of closed head injuries is reviewed; both short- and long-term outcome studies of recovery are examined. A brief review of rehabilitation for the pediatric patient is also presented. Wherever possible, recent advances in our knowledge of the behavioral effects of head trauma are presented. The concluding section suggests directions for future research.

Epidemiology of Pediatric Head Injuries

Several studies have attempted to estimate the incidence of traumatic brain injuries for the general population, including the pediatric age group (Annegers, 1983; Guyer & Ellers, 1990; Hahn et al., 1988; Ivan, Choo, & Ventureya, 1983; Kraus, 1987; Kraus, Fife, Cox, Ramstein, & Conroy, 1986). Rates vary according to criteria for reporting the type and the severity of injury (Kraus, 1987; Kraus, Rock, & Hemyari, 1990), yielding estimates ranging from 193/100,000 to 367/100,000 persons per year for the United States. When rates are adjusted by age, estimates yield a peak incidence for persons aged 15 to 24 years, with secondary peaks observed for infants and young children and for the elderly. Beyond infancy and early childhood, sex differences are observed in the incidence of head injuries, with males preferentially affected over females in a ratio of 2:1. Kraus et al. report that "rates for males increase slowly after age 5 years and increase dramatically at ages 15 and 19 years, while rates for females decline after age 3, rising only moderately after age 12 years" (1990, p. 685). To illustrate, for example, in the year 1981 in San Diego County, California, there were 185/100,000 injuries to males 15 years or younger compared to 132/100,000 for females. Race differences have also been observed with blacks (and other nonwhites) showing a higher rate than whites, although the rate for Hispanic groups is still controversial (Cooper, Tabaddor, & Hauser, 1983; Kraus, 1987; Rivara & Mueller, 1986). However, studies of racial or ethnic differences in the rate of head injuries often fail to calculate the effects of socioeconomic status on the incidence estimates. Kraus (1987) reviewed 10 major incidence studies and observed that the highest brain injury rates were observed in those groups with the lowest median income. Severity estimates (Kraus et al., 1990) suggest that for children aged 0 to 15 years, 5% of brain injuries are fatal, 6% are rated as severe, 8% are reported as of moderate severity, and 82% are mild. Finally, it should be noted that the majority of incidence estimates are based upon hospital admission data or upon emergency room visits, which may yield lower incidence estimates for children who have sustained minor brain trauma (Levin, Ewing-Cobbs, & Fletcher, 1989), especially if they are victims of child abuse (Menkes & Batzdorf, 1974; Rutter, Chadwick, & Shaffer, 1984; Shapiro, 1987). In this latter group, characterized in a recent review (Christoffel, 1990) as victims of "intentional" (vs. accidental) injuries, are included children who sustain abuse from caretakers, siblings, and noncaretakers. Current estimates suggest that the number of child abuse and neglect cases reported has increased about 200% in recent years, with rates ranging from 6.3/1000 cases ages 0 to 2 years to 27.5/1000 cases ages 15 to 17 (Christoffel, 1990).

Causes of Pediatric Head Trauma

There are substantial differences between children and adults in the settings in which head injuries occur (Annegers, 1983; Luerssen, Klauber, & Marshall, 1988; Menkes & Batzdorf, 1974; Rutter et al., 1984; Shapiro, 1987). In infancy and early childhood, the major causes of head injuries include falls in the home, falls in the play area, pedestrian–motor vehicle accidents, bicycle–motor vehicle accidents, sports activities, and child abuse. By the adolescent years, the major causes of head injuries shift predominantly to injuries sustained in motor vehicle accidents, followed by injuries sustained in recreational and sports activities. Kraus (1987) noted some seasonal variation in the causes of head trauma, with bicycle-related accidents peaking in the spring and summer months. A relationship between the cause of injury and its severity has also been observed, with motor vehicle–related accidents more likely to yield more severe injuries and a higher number of fatal injuries (Kraus, 1987; Menkes & Batzdorf, 1984; Shapiro, 1987). For example, motor vehicle accidents account for approximately 10.5% of deaths in children aged 1 to 4 years and 8.9% of deaths for those between 5 and 14 years of age.

Recent research has been devoted to better identification of children who are at greater risk for injuries as well as to the development of better educational programs to prevent injuries. For example, Speltz, Gonzales, Sulzbacher, and Quan (1990) have developed and presented preliminary validity data on the Injury Behavior Checklist, a parent report measure. The checklist consists of 24 "risky" behaviors for children in the preschool ages (e.g., plays carelessly or recklessly, stands on chairs). It was found to distinguish significantly between children with one or no injuries and children with two or more injuries over a varying follow-up period. Profiles of children at risk for injuries due to abuse or neglect have also been developed from national data (Christoffel, 1990); they include young maternal age, unwanted pregnancy, family history of childhood disturbances, foster care, and poverty and its consequences. Similar profiles of risk factors for assault and homicide among adolescent males and females also are available (Christoffel, 1990). Prevention programs that go beyond state law–mandated child car seats, motorcycle helmets, and use of seat belts are being developed. For example, the National Highway Traffic Safety Administration (Washington, DC) has developed school pedestrian safety programs that focus on preventing children from darting into traffic or running across intersections. Instructional parent training programs have been developed to help parents decrease risky or dangerous behaviors in young children (Dershewitz & Williamson, 1984; Mathews, Friman, Barone, Ross, & Christophersen, 1987). Because estimates of the incidence of use of protective helmets are as low as between 1% and 5% of those who bicycle, community programs such as Seattle's Children's Bicycle Helmet campaign aim to increase parental support for children's bicycle helmet use, reduce the costs of purchasing a helmet, and educate children to overcome their reluctance to wear bicycle helmets. Finally, prevention of childhood injuries recently has been declared to be a major priority among health care professionals including pediatricians, neurosurgeons, psychologists, nurses, and child care workers. This follows publication of a Report to Congress prepared by the Center for Disease Control, in Atlanta, Georgia (*Congressional Record*, October 1989).

Table 2.1. Types of head injuries.

Penetrating head injuries	Nonpenetrating head injuries
Depressed skull fractures	Linear skull fractures
Missile (perforation) injury	Closed head injuries

Types of Traumatic Head Injuries

Trauma to the head does not always produce a brain injury (Boll, 1983). When trauma is sufficient to cause central nervous system insult, a spectrum of disorders may be observed ranging from mild concussion to sustained coma or persistent vegetative state (Table 2.1). Two broad classes of brain trauma can occur: penetrating injuries and nonpenetrating injuries. Penetrating injuries occur when a foreign object strikes the head with sufficient force to cause the skull to fracture and move downward, either tearing the dura or lacerating the brain. A second type of penetrating injury occurs when a missile (e.g., a bullet) passes through the skull and dura, lodging in or passing through the brain tissue (perforating injury). Nonpenetrating injuries occur when the force of trauma to the head results in a nondepressed skull fracture (e.g., linear fracture) or when, in the absence of a frank fracture, the force of the trauma is transmitted to the brain within the skull vault. This second class of injuries subsumes the broad group of so-called closed head traumas (Fletcher & Levin, 1988; Levin, Benton, & Grossman, 1982).

In penetrating injuries to the brain, both focal and diffuse effects of the trauma may be observed (Table 2.2). Focal tears in the dura, subsequent injuries to the vessels supplying the dura or the meninges, focal contusions, and/or tearing of brain tissue underlying the depressed skull

Table 2.2. Types of brain injuries following penetrating and nonpenetrating head trauma.

Focal effects—primary

A. Penetrating brain injuries
   1. Tearing dura
   2. Tearing of surface vasculature, epidural or subdural bleeds
   3. Focal compression/laceration of brain tissue
   4. Intracranial contusions (coup or contrecoup)
   5. Intracranial hemorrhage
   6. Focal fragments or trajectory lesions to brain tissue

B. Nonpenetrating brain injuries
   1. Intracranial contusions (coup or contrecoup)
   2. Tearing of surface vasculature
   3. Intracranial hemorrhage

Diffuse effects of brain trauma of either type

A. Primary
   1. Axonal shearings/stretching

B. Secondary
   1. Cerebral edema
   2. Diffuse brain swelling
   3. Increased intracranial pressure
   4. Focal edema surrounding focal traumatic or hemorrhagic lesions
   5. Ischemic brain damage due to blood loss or cardiac or respiratory disorders
   6. Axonal degeneration
   7. Posttraumatic hydrocephalus

fragment and/or other focal tearing of tissue, including pathway lesions and lesions arising from skull fragments penetrating brain tissue, can be observed from perforating missile injuries to the brain (Menkes & Batzdorf, 1974; Shapiro, 1987). Diffuse effects of the mechanical trauma to the head, such as neuronal stretching and shearing and periventricular injuries, as well as contrecoup contusions may also occur in penetrating brain injuries.

Closed head injuries result in brain injury because of the forces transmitted by the initial compression of the head against an object as well as the effects of the resultant acceleration–deceleration movement on the brain contents within the skull. The initial impact of a moving head upon a slower moving or stationary object causes the sudden deceleration of the skull, and the brain may move forward, backward, or side-to-side within the skull vault. Such linear or rotational movements of the brain can lead to blunt trauma to the surfaces of the brain as it impacts on the bony protuberances of the inner skull, particularly in the frontal regions and over the temporal poles, both at the site of impact (coup) and opposite to the point of impact (contrecoup). These same movements can also stretch and tear nerve axons, leading to diffuse axonal injury including periventricular pathway lesions. Blood vessels may be torn or ruptured by these linear or rotational forces, resulting in collections of blood above the dura (epidural hematoma), below the dura (subdural hematoma), or within the brain tissue itself (intracranial hematoma). Brain contusions most often are associated with depressed skull fractures in children; epidural and subdural hematomas are less common in children (below the age of 15) than in adults (Shapiro, 1987).

A number of secondary effects of head trauma also may occur. These can include hypoxia, shock, seizures, and elevated intracranial pressure (ICP) due to diffuse brain swelling or cerebral edema in response to the presence of intracranial hematomas or contused brain tissue. Children, unlike adults, are at greater risk to develop diffuse cerebral swelling following a brain injury. Estimates suggest that 29% of conscious head injured children and 40% of comatose children show evidence of diffuse cerebral swelling on cerebral axial tomography (CT) scan (Shapiro, 1987). For this reason, ICP is now monitored routinely (Mickle, 1989). Children also are more prone to develop seizures in the immediate postinjury period than are adults, although the overall incidence of posttraumatic epilepsy is low (2.5%). Interestingly, children appear more likely than adults to experience early posttraumatic seizures after minor head trauma (Jennett, 1975) but do not appear to be at greater risk to develop late posttraumatic epilepsy (Annegers et al., 1980). Another late effect of diffuse injury, white matter degeneration, has been described in the pediatric age group as well as in adults (Graham, Adams, & Gennarelli, 1987). White matter degeneration is thought to result from retraction of axonal pathways following injury.

In its mildest form, a closed head injury may result in concussion which causes a momentary alteration or disruption in neurologic functioning (Gennarelli, 1987). Consciousness is preserved but there may be a brief period of confusion or disorientation. In classical concussion, there is an alteration of consciousness for a period of up to 6 hours following head trauma. Typically, this is accompanied by other signs of neurologic disorder, including bradycardia, blood pressure changes, changes in muscle tone and/or pupillary responses, and amnesia (Gennarelli, 1987). In children, a delayed onset of central nervous system (CNS) signs has been described (childhood concussion syndrome). In these cases, the child may appear stunned following a head trauma but there is no clear loss of consciousness, and ongoing activities are resumed. Minutes to hours later, pallor, nausea, vomiting, and irritability develop; the child recovers fully from these symptoms within 24 hours (Shapiro, 1987). Postconcussion symptoms described in children and adolescents include headaches, irritability, lethargy, emotional lability, neurovegetative disturbances, memory disorder, and, academic difficulties (Casey, Ludwig, & McCormick, 1986; Lanser, Jennekens-Schinkel, & Peters, 1988; Levin et al., 1989). Compared to studies of the adult postconcussion syndrome (Rutherford, 1989), there has been little research on the incidence, severity, and time course of the resolution of these symptoms in the pediatric age group. This relative paucity of data is troubling given recent estimates of the incidence of mild head trauma in the child and adolescent population, which suggest that almost 88% of children aged 14 years or younger who suffer a head injury will sustain a minor or mild trauma including the spectrum of concussion diagnoses (Levin et al., 1989).

Age Effects in Recovery from Head Injury

In the following sections we review those studies that examined the neuropsychological and neurobehavioral consequences of closed head injury in children and adolescents. As Shapiro (1987) notes, injury to a child's brain affects a system in which neuronal development, myelination, and biochemical reactions related to brain maturation are ongoing processes. As a result, an insult to the developing brain may yield different effects depending upon the level of functional maturity attained at the time of injury as well as upon the yet-to-be developed functional abilities. Thus age-dependent differences may be observed in loss or alteration of function as well as in recovery from injury (Fletcher et al., 1987).

At least three different positions have been offered regarding age effects in injury and recovery from brain damage (Fletcher & Levin, 1988; Taylor, 1984): (1) children show greater vulnerability and less recovery of function than adults; (2) children show greater behavioral sparing and recovery from head injury than adults; and (3) the effects of brain injury in children will depend upon the age of the child, and recovery from injury will depend upon the potential of the immature brain to develop alternative behavioral strategies. In general, studies of the effects of pediatric head injuries and of outcome depend upon the ability of the investigators to classify initial injury severity and specify outcome criteria.

Earlier pediatric studies assessed severity of injury on the basis of the extent of loss of consciousness, presence of skull fracture or hematoma, and accompanying focal or diffuse neurological abnormalities. More recent studies have relied upon the Glascow Coma Scale (Teasdale & Jennett, 1974) for older children (age 3 and above) and the Children's Coma Scale (Hahn et al., 1988) for younger (preschool age and below) children (Table 2.3). Recent development of this standardized scale for infants, toddlers, and younger aged children is a notable advance in the ability of epidemiologists and health care professionals to obtain better comparability across studies of head injuries in younger children. If experience with the Glascow Coma Scale is borne out in this newer scale, greater cooperation between trauma and rehabilitation centers may expand our knowledge of this younger age group. Similarly, earlier studies of recovery of function and outcome frequently relied upon global clinical ratings, whereas more recent studies have applied more systematic assessment techniques such as the Glascow Outcome Scale. Unfortunately, this measure is of limited utility except for the oldest

Table 2.3. Glascow coma scale (GCS) and children's coma scale (CCS) (maximum score = 15).

Eye openings (GCS, CCS)	Best motor response (GCS, CCS)
4. Spontaneous	6. Responds to verbal commands
3. Nonspecific reaction to speech	5. Localized movement to terminate painful stimulus
2. Response to painful stimulus	4. Withdrawal from painful stimulus
1. No response	3. Decorticate posture
	2. Decerebrate posture
	1. No response
Best verbal response (GCS)	**Best behavioral response (CCS)**
5. Oriented	5. Smiles, oriented to sound, interacts, follows objects
4. Confusion, disorientation	4. Consolable crying, but inappropriate interactions
3. No sustained or coherent conversation	3. Inconsistently consolable, moaning
2. No recognizable words	2. Inconsolable, restless, and irritable
1. No response	1. No response

Note: Modified and adapted from "Assessment of Coma and Impaired Consciousness: A Practical Scale" by G. Teasdale and B. Jennett, 1972, *Lancet*, *2*, pp. 81–84, and "Head Injuries in Children Under 36 Months of Age" by Y. S. Hahn, C. Chyung, M. J. Barthel, J. Bailes, A. Flannery, and D. G. McLone, 1988, *Child's Nervous System*, *4*, pp. 34–40.

group of adolescent patients and does not include direct assessment of cognitive or emotional symptoms. For most pediatric patients, outcome continues to be defined by school attendance, school performance, and parental report of cognitive and emotional symptoms.

Studies also differ in the time interval from injury to initial assessment or to outcome assessment as well as whether same-aged control or contrast groups are used. For example, there are relatively few studies comparing mildly head injured children to age-matched normal controls and very few that compare the effects of minor trauma to mild trauma. Despite this, neuropsychologists are often expected to make prognostic statements regarding the long-range outcome from such injuries. Finally, studies differ in the types of tests used to assess the behavioral sequelae of head injury and in the scope and depth of the assessments employed. Despite these difficulties, a number of findings have emerged regarding the effects of head trauma in pediatric patients. These findings begin to depict a more accurate picture of the potential changes in behavior which can occur following head injuries in children and adolescents. In the following sections we review the findings related to intellectual functions, attentional functions, memory, language, motor functions, achievement and academic performance, and behavioral/psychiatric disorders.

Intellectual Functions

A number of investigators have reported declines in scores on standardized tests of intelligence following head trauma. For example, Klonoff, Low, and Clark (1977) reported that initial Full Scale IQ (FSIQ) scores in a group of 231 children between ages 2.7 and 15 years with mild, moderate, or severe head injuries were significantly below those of an age-matched normal control group. Chadwick, Rutter, Shaffer, and Shrout (1981) found that the baseline Verbal (VIQ), Performance (PIQ), and Full Scale (FSIQ) IQ scores of 28 head injured children (mean age 10.03 years) were below those of a matched control group of orthopedically injured boys (mean age 10.12 years). At initial assessment, the mean IQ scores for the head injured group was 96.1 ± 16.0 versus 106.4 ± 13.2 for the orthopedic controls. The mean PIQ for the head injured group was 76.8 ± 21.8 compared to 107.0 ± 18.5 for the orthopedic control group. Levin and Eisenberg (1979a) compared median IQ scores between mild ($n = 8$), moderate ($n = 5$), and severely ($n = 17$) injured children and adolescents at initial entry into a head injury treatment facility. Severity of injury appeared most related to PIQ scores, with the lowest median PIQ (95) obtained by children in the severe head group. The severe group also showed the largest decline from estimates of premorbid intellectual levels. Slater and Bassett (1988) reported that mean FSIQ scores, VIQ scores, and PIQ scores of 33 teenagers who sustained closed head injury were significantly below those obtained by age-matched orthopedically injured and normal control groups in the immediate posttraumatic period. More recently, Bassett and Slater (1990) observed that mildly head injured pediatric patients demonstrated significant VIQ, PIQ, and FSIQ discrepancies from age-matched normal controls as early as 2 months postinjury. Taken together, these studies suggest that pediatric head injury patients experience deficits in FSIQ and PIQ relative to both normal and non–head injured control groups. Deficits in VIQ are not always observed. A number of clinical speculations about these findings have been offered. Most suggest that with the exception of two verbal subtests which are timed or depend heavily upon attention and concentration (Arithmetic, Digit Span), the remainder of the VIQ subtests depend upon old learning or more remotely learned material which is more resistant to change resulting from organic pathology (Boll, 1983). Thus the extent of these VIQ–PIQ differences appears to be most related to the severity of the head injury as indexed by neurologic criteria (Klonoff et al., 1977) or the Glasgow Coma Scale (GCS) (Slater & Bassett, 1988).

The length of follow-up studies assessing intellectual changes following closed head injuries in pediatric patients has ranged from 6 months to 5 years. For example, Levin and Eisenberg (1979b) found that VIQ and PIQ deficits were commonly seen in patients with severe head injuries at follow-up intervals of 4 to 8 months. Similarly, Levin, Eisenberg, Wigg, and Kobayashi (1982) reported lower median VIQ and PIQ scores in patients with GCS scores of 8 or less (i.e., the more severely injured) when seen an average of 6 months posttrauma. In contrast, when comparing 56 mildly head injured children to a grade-, age-, and sex-matched control group of normal children, Gulbrandsen (1984) reported no significant difference in VIQ (101.4 ± 11.7), PIQ (109.9 ± 12.7), or FSIQ (106.0 ± 11.4) when assessed at 6 months posttrauma. Comparing mildly and moderately injured younger and older children to severely injured children in the same age ranges, Bassett and Slater (1990) found deficits at 2 months follow-up and Ewing-Cobbs, Miner, Perkins, and Levin (1989) observed persistent deficits for the severely injured group at 6 months following injury. For more severely injured children, persistent differences in FSIQ (Klonoff et al., 1977) or PIQ (Chadwick et al., 1981) have also been reported at 1 year follow-up when brain injured children are compared to a control group of normal children or orthopedically injured children.

Among brain injured pediatric patients, the degree of injury (mild, moderate, severe) appears to be related to longer term outcome. For example, Winogron, Knights, and Bawden (1984) reported the persistence of PIQ deficits only for the group of severely injured children at 1 year follow-up. These same children were reported in a subsequent study (Bawden, Knights, & Winogron, 1985) to show VIQ scores (86.6 ± 17.6), PIQ scores (80.1 ± 24.1), and FSIQ scores (82.1 ± 21.5) falling in the Low Average to Borderline ranges. Similarly, Berger-Gross and Shackelford (1985) reported that 6.7% of their subjects showed deficient IQ scores 1 year after their head injury. Studies involving lengthier follow-up periods also support the observation that severely brain injured children may experience persistent IQ deficits at $2\frac{1}{2}$ years (Chadwick et al., 1981), 3 years (Filley, Cranberg, Alexander, & Hart, 1987), 4 years (Mahoney et al., 1983), and 5 years from the initial insult in both younger and older head injured patients (Klonoff et al., 1977). These findings are consistent with earlier studies of mixed types of severely injured children (Black, Blumer, Wellner, & Walker, 1971; Brink, Garrett, Hall, Woo-Sam, & Nickle, 1970; Heiskanen & Kaste, 1974).

However, these findings must be interpreted with caution, particularly when clinicians are asked to evaluate the long-term outcome of head injury in the individual case. A particular problem is the differential attrition rate in longitudinal studies of head injured children. For example, it is unclear what percentage of children with fewer residual deficits are lost to follow-up resulting in a preponderance of children with greater deficits in longitudinal studies. Similarly, given the current epidemiological data on childhood head injuries, the population of mildly injured children is clearly underrepresented in available studies. Finally, virtually no larger scale collaborative studies have attempted to control for (or often even to report) the possible confounding effects of such factors as socioeconomic status on premorbid estimates of intellectual abilities. Available evidence does support the likelihood that severely head injured children will show deficits on standardized intelligence tests for periods of up to 5 years postinjury. Age at time of injury does not appear to be related to these outcomes.

Attentional Functions

Attentional disorders following closed head injuries have been reported widely for adult patients suffering the full spectrum of injury severity ranging from concussion (Binder, 1986; Rutherford, 1989) to recovery from extended coma (Levin, Eisenberg, et al., 1982; Levin, Grafman, & Eisenberg, 1987). Estimates of attentional disorder have been based upon a variety of information sources. These sources included observational data on patient behavior, patient reports, and performance on tests designed to directly assess attention. Parental and teacher reports are additional sources of information for the pediatric head injured group.

Early studies of severely injured children (Black, Jeffries, Blumer, Wellner, & Walker, 1969; Bruce, Schut, Bruno, Wood, & Sutton, 1978) reported the presence of attentional disorder symptoms at follow-up periods from 1 to 7 years after injury. Most commonly, hyperactivity and short attention span were reported by parents at follow-up examinations (Brink et al., 1970). Klonoff et al. (1977) found that younger head injured children (less than 9 years old) showed deficits on neuropsychological tests of response speed and accuracy as well as in parental reports of problems in attention and concentration compared to controls up to 5 years postinjury. Differences between older injured children and controls were not observed beyond 2 years postinjury. Klonoff et al. (1977) do not specifically interpret this observed age effect with regard to attention complaints except to note the markedly larger variances observed within the head injured groups compared to controls. This observation certainly supports the often stated dictum in clinical neuropsychology that brain injury usually results in greater variability in behavior.

Similar residual deficits in attention were also reported by parents of 50% of pediatric multisystem trauma patients at 1 year follow-up (Harris, Schwaitzberg, Seman, & Herrmann, 1989). Even children who sustained mild head trauma have demonstrated deficits compared to controls on neuropsychological measures sensitive to attention at 6 months postinjury (Gulbrandsen, 1984), although the group differences observed were not significant when age was factored into the analyses. Winogron and colleagues (Bawden et al., 1985; Winogron et al., 1984) observed deficits on tests dependent upon concentration and speeded performance for mildly, moderately, and severely injured children at 1 year posttrauma. In contrast, Chadwick et al. (1981) reported that performance on a continuous performance test and a test of behavioral impulsivity improved between initial assessment and 1 year follow-up for a group of severely head injured children. Parental reports of newly observed problems in social inappropriateness, hyperectivity, and impulsivity persisted throughout the $2\frac{1}{2}$ year follow-up period among severly injured children. These symptoms were interpreted to be similar to the frontal lobe syndromes observed in adults with severe head injuries (Rutter et al., 1984). Recently, Fletcher and colleagues (1990) challenged this interpretation except among severely head injured children. Comparing parental reports of adaptive skills and problem behaviors at 6 month and 1 year follow-up, these authors found a greater association between cognitive and behavioral outcome only up to 1 year follow-up.

Review of these studies seems to support the conclusion that severe head injury frequently results in persistent problems in attention. Unfortunately, again, the limits of available data are evident. A major drawback to current studies is the difficulty in correlating behavioral data, performance on tests thought to assess attention, and parental or teacher report of problem behaviors which are observed at home or in the classroom. This problem emerges from at least two sources: (1) the disparity between the broad conceptual domain of attention and its narrower definition on such clinical tests as digit span, continuous performance tests, or simple and choice reaction time tasks; and (2) the lack of agreement between specific behavioral report measures such as problem checklists and various neuropsychological measures. Research with pediatric head injured patients clearly is in need of the type of construct validation efforts of attentional measures recently reported by Shum, McFarland, and Bain (1990) among adult head injured patients and normals. These authors identified three major factors among 8 attention tasks: visuomotor scanning; sustained selective processing, and visual/auditory spanning.

The task for child neuropsychologists is a formidable one, however, given the differential maturation of brain systems related to attention arousal and response initiation as well as differential maturation in those systems related to language and verbally guided behavior (self-talk). Furthermore, it is important to remind clinicians that even among moderately and severely head injured children, there is a lack of uniformity in the behavioral complaints and performance deficits observed. It is also unclear whether there is a significant modification in the clinical picture with increasing age, although early reports suggest significant improvement over time (Klonoff et al., 1977). Finally, there is a clear lack of instruments developed to specifically address the spectrum of attention problems which can follow head injury, including indices of both frequency of problem behaviors (i.e., hyperactivity) and intensity (i.e., how troubling to the parent/teacher), such as have been developed for conduct disordered children (Robinson, Eyberg, & Ross, 1980). It is hoped that proposed revisions to the American Psychiatric Association's classification of childhood behavior problems (DSM IV) will clarify the variety of attentional disorders which can be observed, including those not accompanied by other behaviors such as hyperactivity and impulsivity.

Memory

Complaints of attention and concentration problems frequently coexist with performance deficits on tests of memory and learning among pediatric head injured patients (Fletcher, Ewing-Cobbs, Miner, Levin, & Eisenberg, 1990; Levin et al., 1982). Evaluating memory deficits in very young patients is problematic given the differences in the strategies employed on memory tasks between younger and older children (Kail, 1982). As a result, comprehensive evaluations of younger head injured patients often do not report memory data (Ewing-Cobbs, Miner, Fletcher, & Levin, 1989), or younger patients are excluded from the study groups (Chadwick et al., 1981). Despite these difficulties, a review of the literature suggests that closed head injuries in the pediatric age group (2 to 15 years) can result in memory disorder. Both nonverbal and verbal memory problems have been observed.

Nonverbal Memory Deficits

Klonoff et al. (1977) reported deficits in memory for shapes and location on the Tactual Performance Test (TPT) in a mixed group of younger and older head injured children. Memory for shapes was impaired at initial evaluation and at 3 year follow-up for the younger children (<9 years), whereas the initial memory deficits observed in older children persisted to only the 1 year follow-up period. Location memory seemed less sensitive, in that differences between head injured children and controls persisted only to 1 year follow-up for the older children and was seen at 1 and 3 year follow-up in the younger children. Similar problems in TPT location have been reported for moderately and severely injured groups at 1 year follow-up by Winogron et al. (1984) but not for mildly head injured children at 6 months posttrauma (Gulbrandsen, 1984). Similarly, Berger-Gross and Shackelford (1985) reported that 20% of their severely head injured patients (mean age 9.2 years) had deficient scores on a visual reproduction memory task at 1 year postcoma. More recently, Bassett and Slater (1990) also reported deficits in immediate and delayed visual reproduction memory among severely head injured adolescents but not for the mildly injured group when compared to age-matched normal controls.

Verbal Memory Deficits

Verbal memory deficits following head trauma have been examined in a series of collaborative studies conducted in Galveston, Texas. For example, Levin and Eisenberg (1979a, 1979b) demonstrated problems in the storage and retrieval of new verbal material (i.e., word lists) among mildly, moderately, and severely head injured children and adolescents at initial evaluation. These differences persisted at 6 month follow-up, although with greater rates of improvement observed in the mildly injured group (Levin, Eisenberg, et al., 1982). In this same study, performance on a visual verbal recognition memory task was also shown to be affected at initial assessment and at 6 month follow-up, but only for the severely injured group. Considerable improvement over baseline testing was observed in the mildly and moderately injured patients. Levin et al. (1988) reported no deficits in verbal memory at initial testing following resolution of posttraumatic amnesia or at 1 year follow-up in a group of mildly and moderately injured children. Severely injured children were impaired at initial and follow-up assessments. Deficits in recognition memory were also observed at initial testing in both groups, but these deficits had resolved by 1 year follow-up for the mild/moderate groups only. In an earlier study, deficits in learning word pairs were observed at initial and 4 month follow-up but not at 1 year posttrauma in a group of severely head injured children ages 5 to 14 (Chadwick et al., 1981). More recently, Bassett and Slater (1990) reported deficits in the immediate and delayed recall of story passages among severely head injured adolescents. Their group of mildly injured patients, however, did not differ from normal controls in either recall condition.

In summary, review of relevant research supports the presence of nonverbal and verbal learning and memory problems among severely head injured children and adolescents. These deficits appear to persist to at least 1 year posttrauma. The findings with regard to mildly and moderately head injured children are less clear. Some investigators report problems in learning word lists and word pairs; others suggest that story recall and digit span are only marginally affected and only for limited periods of follow-up study. Disentangling specific problems in memory processing such as encoding versus retrieval from problems in attention and concentration continues to be needed in studies of children with head injuries. Studies of various parameters of memory performance and adequate normative data for different age groups are still needed in child neuropsychology (Fennell & Bauer, 1989). Future research should include memory tasks designed to evaluate information processing models of memory in head injured children, which may allow for better description of memory dysfunction in these patients.

Efforts to relate the nature of memory deficits to focus of lesion have yielded mixed results. Rutter et al. (1984) reported no consistent laterality or locus effects in the patterns of cognitive deficits following brain injury. This position is consistent with other views of lateralized findings in children with brain lesions (Boll & Barth, 1981). Recent studies employing magnetic resonance imaging (MRI) have demonstrated that some brain contusions may be missed or underestimated in size utilizing conventional CT scans (Snow, Zimmerman, Gandy, & Deck, 1986; Wilberger, Deeb, & Rothfus, 1987). In particular, lesions involving the frontotemporal regions appear to be better visualized when an MRI is employed. Levin, Amparo, Eisenberg, Williams, High, McArdle, and Weiner (1987) recently reported a relationship between the size and location of MRI lesions and deficits on tests of frontal lobe functioning and memory in a group of 20 adult head injured patients. Improvements in cognitive functioning at 1 month and 3 month follow-up testing were paralleled by changes in the MRI lesion findings. These results suggest that future research employing MRI in closed head injured patients may provide greater diagnostic concordance between behavioral and laboratory data as well as a foundation for understanding the course of recovery of function. More studies of the relationship between MRI lesions and behavioral disorders, including memory deficits, in the pediatric age group are clearly needed. In particular, longitudinal studies of MRI lesions among pediatric head injured patients could begin to correlate deficits in maturation of behaviors with persistent areas of focal damage as well as potentially monitor the emergence of trauma-related structural anomalies.

Language

A rather narrow spectrum of speech and language disorders has been described following head injuries in the pediatric age group. Early reports on acquired aphasia in children rarely attributed the disorder to head injury (Alajouanine & Lhermitte, 1965; Hecaen, 1976). However, recent reviews suggest that speech and language disturbances following head trauma can include mutism, motor speech disturbances, and frank aphasias, as well as a variety of more subtle alterations in language functions (i.e., aphasoid symptoms) involving naming, word retrieval, and deficits in written language and comprehension (Ylvisaker, 1986). Mutism following head trauma is more commonly observed in younger children and is typically followed by gradual resolution (Hecaen, 1976). Estimates of the initial incidence and persistence of aphasic disorders vary from study to study. For example, early studies (Brink et al., 1970) reported that articulation defects were observed in 20/46 severely injured pediatric patients, with an additional 6 patients showing varying degrees of expressive aphasia. Estimates from more recent studies range from 63.1% of a group of 84 severely head injured young persons (Gilchrist & Wilkinson, 1979) to between 31% and 35% of pediatric closed head injury patients (Kaiser & Pfenninger, 1984; Levin & Eisenberg, 1979a, 1979b). When severity of injury is examined, the incidence of language disorder escalates with increasing severity (Levin & Eisenberg, 1979a, 1979b). Although age effects on the incidence of language disorders have yielded mixed findings, a recent study of head injured children and adolescents (Ewing-Cobbs, Fletcher, Levin, & Landry, 1985) suggests that age effects are related to the skills that are in development at the time of the injury. For example, relatively greater vulnerability to written language disturbances was observed for the younger children but not for the adolescents.

Direct assessment of language functions in head injured children and adolescents has documented problems in object naming (Chadwick et al., 1981; Jordan, Ozanne, & Murdoch, 1990; Levin & Eisenberg, 1979a, 1979b), verbal fluency (Chadwick et al., 1981; Slater & Bassett, 1988; Winogron et al., 1984), repetition (Levin & Eisenberg, 1979a, 1979b), written language tasks (Ewing-Cobbs, Levin, Eisenberg, & Fletcher, 1987), and motor speech/articulation disorders (Filley et al., 1987). Younger children (below age 5 years) reportedly manifest problems on both expressive and receptive language measures (Ewing-Cobbs et al., 1987) at initial evaluation. At follow-up, children with severe head injury continued to function below the mild/moderate group, despite improvements from baseline levels. The initial finding of impairments in expressive language for all age groups was not observed by 9 months postinjury.

In most studies of language functioning in head injured children, the follow-up period has typically ranged from 4 months to 1 year postinjury.

Whether this same pattern of overt and subtle language deficits would be observed over longer follow-up periods remains to be determined in future longitudinal studies. In addition, the evaluations for speech and language deficits are typically presented in the absence of other findings relating to intellectual functions or other neuropsychological functions such as memory, attention, and motor deficits. As a result, it is not always clear whether the deficits reported appear as part of a constellation of problems following brain injury or could be confounded by other deficits (e.g., memory). Furthermore, there has been no substantial effort to relate CT or MRI data on focal lesions to the pattern of language problems observed. Future research efforts which control for these factors (larger studies, CT and MRI lesion location, co-occurring neuropsychological deficits, and longitudinal outcome) are needed. Until such time, clinicians may be wise to limit their conclusions to descriptive studies of these children and adolescents.

Motor Functions

The majority of studies that have addressed the integrity of motor functions following closed head injuries have relied upon descriptions of motor abnormalities observed on the neurologic examination (Shapiro, 1987). Fewer studies have utilized direct assessment of motor performance on a variety of tasks which evaluate fine motor speed (e.g., finger tapping) or manual dexterity (e.g., grooved pegboard). Other investigators have evaluated motor performance using tasks that depend upon speeded visuomotor or tactual motor performance (e.g., Tactual Performance Test).

Motor slowing appears to be a prominent feature of the initial period following mild, moderate, and severe head injury (Levin, Benton, et al., 1982). However, several studies suggest that children who are severely injured are at greater risk for residual motor speed or dexterity deficits at 6 months (Levin & Eisenberg, 1979a, 1979b), 1 year (Bawden et al., 1985; Chadwick et al., 1981; Winogron et al., 1984), and 2 years of follow-up (Klonoff et al., 1977). In contrast, mildly head injured children examined at 6 months postinjury did not differ from a normal control group on speed of finger tapping (Gulbrandsen, 1984).

Skills that depend upon integrating motor performance with perceptual functioning have also been examined. For example, impairments in fine visuomotor copying skills and visuomotor constructional abilities have been directly measured (Bawden et al., 1985; Chadwick et al., 1981; Klonoff et al., 1977; Levin & Eisenberg, 1979a, 1979b) or inferred from analysis of the performance subtests of standard intelligence tests such as the Wechsler scales (Fletcher & Levin, 1988). Focal neurological signs of motor dysfunction such as hemiparesis, ataxia, or facial weakness have typically been employed to document motor deficits in those large-scale studies that depended upon global severity ratings at initial assessment or at outcome (Alberico, Ward, Choi, Marmarou, & Young, 1987; Hahn et al., 1988; Ivan et al., 1983).

Studies reviewed suggest that deficits in elementary motor functions as well as problems on tasks which depend upon speed, accuracy, or dexterity can follow head injuries in children and adolescents. Here again, the absence of sophisticated lesion location studies utilizing consecutive MRI scans as well as the absence of longitudinal studies limits the generalizations one can draw from these studies to the individual case, particularly regarding recovery of function. Future studies may need to address these deficiencies.

Achievement and Academic Performance

Persistent problems in academic performance following pediatric head injury have been reported in a number of studies (Ewing-Cobbs et al., 1985; Fletcher & Levin, 1988; Levin et al., 1989). These problems include reading and written language disabilities and arithmetic disabilities. Failure to return to previous grade placement, the need for special educational programs, and failure to return to school appeared in earlier reports of studies of severely head injured children (e.g., Brink et al., 1970; Klonoff et al., 1977). There are fewer studies of children who suffer mild or moderate brain injuries.

Given the findings of language problems in preschool-age as well as school-age mildly and moderately injured children, it would not be surprising that difficulties might ensue when the child enters or returns to school. As Ewing-Cobbs et al. (1985) and others suggest, age effects may be a critical factor in the development of different types of learning disabilities. For example, deficits in the acquisition of basic reading skills (e.g., phonics) may be more apparent in the primary grades, whereas problems in reading comprehension, reading speed, and composition may be manifested more in later school grades, which demand these skills. Further, Levin and Benton (1986) reported postinjury decrements in arithmetic performance from preinjury levels in children with mild/moderate or severe closed head injuries. Whether these deficits are a function of problems with reading word problems, with memorizing mathematical procedures, or due to spatial deficits is not clear. Berger-Gross and Shackleford (1985) found that 1 year after severe closed head injury, 6.7% of their small sample of elementary school–age subjects demonstrated a spelling deficiency, one dimension of a written language disorder. An earlier study of reading disability subsequent to depressed skull fractures estimated that 55% of the children were reading at least 1 year below age levels (Shaffer, Bijur, Chadwick, & Rutter, 1980). Unfortunately, the percentage of these children who were behind in reading at the time of the injury was not reported. Of interest, there were no sex differences in the incidence of intermediate or severe reading disability following the skull fracture. This finding is in contrast to the expectation of a preponderance of males who are diagnosed as reading impaired.

Future studies of academic disabilities and achievement deficits in pediatric head injured patients will need to disentangle the confounding influences of premorbid abilities, specific versus generalized learning disabilities, and the effects of memory and attentional disorders on school performance. At present, available empirical and clinical data suggest that reading, mathematics, and written language deficits may follow from moderate to severe closed head injuries. Data with regard to mild injuries remain unclear. The clinician who is assessing a child for academic deficits following head trauma will need to carefully review all available achievement assessments which antedate and follow the head trauma.

Behavioral/Psychiatric Disorders

A number of studies suggest that behavior problems may be present in the initial period following even minor head trauma in children. For example, Casey et al. (1986) found that parents of children followed up 1 month after minor head trauma reported changes in temperament and in school attendance. Studies of children with mild to moderate head injuries (Rutter et al., 1984) suggest that although transient symptoms of behavior disorder may be present initially, mild head injury was not associated with an increased incidence of psychiatric disturbances (Gulbransen, 1984; Levin et al., 1989). In contrast, severe head injury frequently results in the development of new behavior disorders (Black et al., 1969; Brink et al., 1970; Filley et al., 1987; Klonoff et al., 1977; Rutter et al., 1984). Estimates of poor social adjustment outcomes from severe head injuries in children have ranged from over 50% at up to 34 months postinjury in the small series of Filley et al. (1987) to about 25% at 1 year follow-up but increasing to about 50% at 5 years follow-up (Klonoff et al., 1977).

Estimates of the incidence of behavioral problems following head trauma may be inflated by the presence of preexisting behavior problems (Rutter et al., 1984), including risk taking behaviors (Speltz et al., 1990). When these confounds are removed, the severely head injured patients still are at greater risk for the development of new psychiatric disorders. Behavior problems which are reported often are nonspecific, such as "personality changes," or can include a variety of specific complaints, such as aggressiveness, hyperactivity, impulsivity, poor social judgment, increased dependency, and the development of fears and phobic disorders. For children with preexisting behavior disorders, posttraumatic changes often consisted of an intensification of the prior problem behaviors. There is a slight incremental effect on the development of new psychiatric disorder among the severely brain injured children if these children also suffer from significant neurological sequelae or intellectual impairment (Fletcher & Levin, 1988; Rutter et al., 1984). Recently, Fletcher et al. (1990) suggested that the major behavior observed in their series of children with severe head injuries included a decline in adaptive behaviors as assessed by the Vineland Adaptive Behavior Scale (Sparrow, Balla, & Chicchetti, 1984) over the 1 year of follow-up postinjury. In addition, the severely head injured children were active in fewer social/school activities. Children with mild injuries did not appear to manifest new behavior problems in the 6 month and 1 year follow-up period.

Review of the foregoing studies suggests that new behavior problems are more likely to follow a severe head injury in children and adolescents as compared to a mild or moderate head injury. In these latter cases, behavior problems have been interpreted to reflect an exacerbation of premorbid problems or transient behavior changes which clear within 3 to 6 months postinjury. A number of limitations are evident, however, in the research cited. Most studies have depended upon parental report of behavior changes obtained at interview or by questionnaire. There have been few efforts to validate these parental reports with school or home observations of behavior problems. The questionnaires employed typically are designed to assess general dimensions of child psychopathology and rarely evaluate the confounding effects of premorbid symptoms, parental concerns, parental stress, changes in parenting behaviors, and academic problems which contribute to the total clinical picture. There have been few prospective longitudinal studies of the evolution of behavior disorder according to age at time of injury and age at follow-up. Those available (e.g., Chadwick et al., 1981; Klonoff et al., 1977) employed broad age groupings, which may not have been sufficiently sensitive to age-maturational effects. More research is needed to assess the specific relationships between cognitive and neuropsychological factors, behavioral symptoms, and neurodiagnostic findings on CT or MRI scans.

Rehabilitation

In contrast to the increasing number of studies of cognitive rehabilitation for adult head injured patients (Benedict, 1989), most studies of treatment of head trauma in pediatric patients have focused on medical management of the acute effects of trauma (Jaffe & Hays, 1986) or of residual posttraumatic disorders such as posttraumatic language disorders. Relatively few children spend extended time as inpatients in a rehabilitation center, particularly children below the age of 6. Younger children commonly are discharged to home/parental care with outpatient rehabilitation care. Postacute admissions to rehabilitation centers often occur in older children needing more intense behavior management and treatment services. Residential rehabilitation programs for children typically include the services of a physical therapist, an occupational therapist, a speech therapist, and a schoolteacher (Jennett & Teasdale, 1981). Depending upon the patient's level of physical disability and speech/language deficits, specific target problems are described and a treatment plan is developed. Thus strengthening weak limbs, designing adaptive feeding devices, and specific articulation therapy may be prescribed to assist the child's recovery.

Unfortunately, there are relatively few empirical studies to guide the development of rehabilitation plans for the kinds of attention, memory, and behavioral/psychiatric disorders that many head injured children manifest (McGuire & Sylvester, 1987; Prigatano et al., 1984). Despite evidence of significant differences between children and adults in problem-solving strategies employed by children, many rehabilitation programs for children are borrowed from adult models (Levin, Grafman, & Eisenberg, 1987) and simply lower the level of performance expected. In the absence of theoretically driven models of cognitive rehabilitation for children (Finger, LeVere, Almli, & Stein, 1988), many clinicians who treat brain injured children must develop a collaborative working relationship with the child's parents and teachers in order to effect environmental changes in the home and school during the course of recovery. Careful assessments are critical to understanding the specific needs of the individual child (Fennell & Bauer, 1989) within his or her family and school setting. The neuropsychologist can play a key role in educating the family and the school about the kinds of processing deficits and problem behaviors experienced by the child recovering from a brain injury. Follow-up neuropsychological and behavioral assessments are also important in order to monitor the changing needs of the recovering child. At present, however, a critical need still exists for carefully controlled empirical studies of the efficacy of current rehabilitation programs for the pediatric age group (see Ylvisaker, Szekeres, & Hartwick, Chapter 6, this volume).

Conclusions

As the preceding review suggests, various behavioral changes can follow trauma to the brain in children and adolescents (Table 2.4). Several themes emerge from the examination of these studies of pediatric head injured patients. First, behavior changes can occur following any type of head trauma, but they do not occur in all instances of trauma. Second, the extent and severity of the behavioral change depend upon the timing of the assessment (e.g., postacute vs. 6 month follow-up). Third, the age at time of trauma influences the pattern of initial behavioral changes as well as the rate and pattern of recovery from these initial deficits and the nature and pattern of persisting deficits. Fourth, the presence of pre-

Table 2.4. Neuropsychological changes following closed head injuries.

Cognitive effects
Declines in Full Scale and Performance IQ scores
Attention/concentration dysfunction
Memory disorder
Language dysfunctions
Motor slowing
Achievement/academic declines
Emotional/behavioral effects
Development of new behavior problems
Exaggeration of preexisting behavior problems

existing problems such as learning disabilities or behavior disorders can influence the pattern and severity of symptoms following head trauma as well as recovery from new behavior disorder. Fifth, greater risk for adverse outcomes is conferred upon children who sustain more severe injuries in contrast to children who are mildly or moderately injured. Finally, the question of whether younger children are more or less vulnerable to adverse outcomes from brain injuries depends upon the functions studied.

These conclusions may require modification as future studies are able to identify with greater accuracy the specific relationships between lesion site and size and neurobehavioral symptoms in the head injured child. In particular, analysis of age-related differences in the nature and extent of behavioral sequelae from brain injury continues to be needed if the clinician is to accurately and sensitively understand the acute and chronic effects of head injuries in children. The same high standards of diagnostic care and rehabilitation now available to adults must be extended to the care of the head injured child. Moreover, continued development of programs of early intervention for injury-prone children and educational efforts to prevent pediatric head injuries should be a national priority for neuropsychologists.

References

Alajouanine, T. H., & Lhermitte, F. (1965). Acquired aphasia in children. *Brain*, *88*, 653–662.

Alberico, A. M., Ward, J. D., Choi, S. C., Marmarou, A., & Young, H. F. (1987). Outcome after severe head injury. *Journal of Neurosurgery*, *67*, 648–656.

Annegers, J. F. (1983). The epidemiology of head trauma in children. In K. Shapiro (Ed.), *Pediatric head trauma* (pp. 1–10). Mount Kisco, NY: Futura Publishing.

Annegers, J. F., Grabow, J. D., Groover, R. V., Laws, E. R., Elveback, L. R., & Kurland, L. T. (1980). Seizure after head trauma: A population study. *Neurology*, *30*, 683–689.

Bassett, S. S., & Slater, E. J. (1990). Neuropsychological function in adolescents sustaining mild closed head injury. *Journal of Pediatric Psychology*, *15*, 225–236.

Bawden, H. N., Knights, R. M., & Winogron, H. W. (1985). Speeded performance following head injury in children. *Journal of Clinical and Experimental Neuropsychology*, *7*, 39–54.

Benedict, R. H. (1989). The effectiveness of cognitive remediation strategies for victims of traumatic head injury: A review of the literature. *Clinical Psychology Review*, *9*, 605–626.

Berger-Gross, P., & Shackelford, M. (1985). Closed head injury in children: Neuropsychological and scholastic outcomes. *Perceptual and Motor Skills*, *61*, 254.

Binder, L. M. (1986). Persisting symptoms after mild head injury: A review of the postconcussive syndrome. *Journal of Clinical and Experimental Neuropsychology*, *8*, 323–346.

Black, P., Blumer, D., Wellner, A. M., & Walker, A. E. (1971). The head-injured child: Time course of recovery with implications for rehabilitation. *Proceeding of an International Symposium on Head Injuries* (pp. 131–137). Edinburgh: Churchill Livingstone.

Black, P. E., Jeffries, J. J., Blumer, D., Wellner, A., & Walker, A. E. (1969). The posttraumatic syndrome in children. In A. M. Walker, W. F. Raveness, & M. Critchley (Eds.). *Late effects of head injury* (pp. 142–149). Springfield, IL: Charles C. Thomas.

Boll, T. M. (1983). Minor head injury in children: Out of sight but not out of mind. *Journal of Clinical and Child Psychology*, *12*, 74–80.

Boll, T. M., & Barth, J. (1981). Neuropsychology of brain damage in children. In S. B. Filskov & T. M. Boll (Eds.), *Handbook of clinical neuropsychology* (Vol. 1, pp. 418–452). New York: Wiley-Interscience.

Brink, J. D., Garrett, A. L., Hale, W. R., Woo-Sam, J., & Nickle, V. L. (1970). Recovery of motor and intellectual function in children sustaining severe head injuries. *Developmental Medicine and Child Neurology*, *12*, 565–571.

Bruce, D. A., Schut, L., Bruno, L. A., Wood, J. H., & Sutton, L. N. (1978). Outcome following severe head injury in children. *Journal of Neurosurgery*, *48*, 679–688.

Casey, R., Ludwig, S., & McCormick, M. C. (1986). Morbidity following minor head trauma in children. *Pediatrics*, *78*, 497–502.

Chadwick, O., Rutter, M., Shaffer, D., & Shrout, P. E. (1981). A prospective study of children with head injuries: IV. Specific cognitive deficits. *Journal of Clinical Neuropsychology*, *3*, 101–120.

Christoffel, K. K. (1990). Violent death and injury in U. S. children and adolescents. *American Journal of Diseases of Children*, *144*, 697–706.

Cooper, J. D., Tabaddor, K., & Hauser, W. A. (1983). The epidemiology of head injury in the Bronx. *Neuroepidemiology*, *2*, 70–88.

Dershewitz, R. A., & Williamson, J. W. (1977). Prevention of childhood household injuries: A controlled clinical trial. *American Journal of Public Health*, *60*, 1148–1153.

Ewing-Cobbs, L., Fletcher, J. M., Levin, H. S., & Landry, S. (1985). Language disorders after pediatric head injury. In J. K. Darby (Ed.), *Speech and language evaluation in neurology, childhood disorders* (pp. 97–112). Orlando, FL: Grune and Stratton.

Ewing-Cobbs, L., Levin, H. S., Eisenberg, H. M., & Fletcher, J. M. (1987). Language functions following closed head injury in children and adolescents. *Journal of Clinical and Experimental Neuropsychology*, *2*, 575–592.

Ewing-Cobbs, L., Miner, M., Fletcher, J. M., & Levin, H. S. (1989). Intellectual, motor and language sequelae following closed head injury in infants and preschoolers. *Journal of Pediatric Psychology*, *14*, 531–547.

Fennell, E. B., & Bauer, R. M. (1989). Models of inference in evaluating brain–behavior relationships in children. In C. R. Reynolds & E. Fletcher-Janzen (Eds.), *Handbook of clinical child neuropsychology* (pp. 167–178). New York: Plenum.

Filley, C. M., Cranberg, L. D., Alexander, M. P., & Hart, E. J. (1987). Neurobehavioral outcome after closed head injury in childhood and adolescence. *Archives of Neurology*, *44*, 194–198.

Finger, S., LeVere, T. E., Almli, R., & Stein, D. G. (1988). *Brain injury and recovery: Theoretical and controversial issues*. New York: Plenum.

Fletcher, J., Ewing-Cobbs, L., Miner, M., Levin, H. S., & Eisenberg, H. M. (1990). Behavioral changes after closed head injury in children. *Journal of Consulting and Clinical Psychology*, *58*, 93–98.

Fletcher, J. M., & Levin, H. S. (1988). Neurobehavioral effects of brain injury in children. In D. K. Routh (Ed.), *Handbook of pediatric psychology* (pp. 258–295). New York: Guilford Press.

Fletcher, J., Miner, M. E., & Ewing-Cobbs, L. (1987). Age and recovery from head injury in children: Developmental issues. In H. S. Levin, J. Grafman, & H. M. Eisenberg (Eds.), *Neurobehavioral recovery from head injury* (pp. 279–291). New York: Oxford University Press.

Gennarelli, T. A. (1987). Cerebral concussion and diffuse brain injuries. In P. R. Cooper (Ed.), *Head injury* (pp. 108–124). Baltimore: Williams & Wilkins.

Gilchrist, E., & Wilkinson, M. (1979). Some factors determining prognosis in young people with severe head injuries. *Archives of Neurology*, *36*, 355–359.

Graham, D. I., Adams, J. H., & Gennarelli, T. A. (1987). Pathology of brain damage in head injury. In P. R. Cooper (Ed.), *Head injury* (pp. 72–88). Baltimore: Williams & Wilkins.

Gulbrandsen, G. B. (1984). Neuropsychological sequelae of light head injuries in older children 6 months after trauma. *Journal of Clinical Neuropsychology*, *6*, 257–268.

Guyer, B., & Ellers, B. (1990). Childhood Injuries in the United States. *American Journal of Disease of Children*, *144*, 649–652.

Hahn, Y. S., Chyung, C., Barthel, M. J., Bailes, J., Flannery, A., & McLone, D. G. (1988). Head injuries in children under 36 months of age. *Child's Nervous System*, *4*, 34–40.

Harris, B. H., Schwaitzberg, S. D., Seman, T. M., & Herrmann, C. (1989). The hidden morbidity of pediatric trauma. *Journal of Pediatric Surgery*, *24*, 103–106.

Hecaen, H. (1976). Acquired aphasia in children and the ontogenesis of hemispheric functional specialization. *Brain and Language*, *3*, 114–134.

Heiskanen, O., & Kaste, M. (1974). Late prognosis of severe brain injury in children. *Developmental Medicine and Child Neurology*, *16*, 11–14.

Ivan, L. F., Choo, S. H., & Ventureya, E. C. (1983). Head injuries in childhood: A 2 year survey. *Canadian Medical Association Journal*, *128*, 281–284.

Jaffe, K. M., & Hays, R. M. (1986). Pediatric head injury: Rehabilitative medical management. *Journal of Head Trauma Rehabilitation*, *4*, 30–40.

Jennett, B. (1975). *Epilepsy after non-missile head injuries*, London: Heinemann.

Jennett, B., & Teasdale, G. (1981). *Management of head injuries*. Philadelphia: F. A. Davis.

Jordan, F. M., Ozanne, A. E., & Murdoch, B. E. (1990). Performance of closed head injured children on a naming task. *Brain Injury*, *4*, 27–32.

Kail, R. (1982). *The Development of Memory in Children*. New York: W. H. Freeman and Company.

Kaiser, G., & Pfenninger, J. (1984). Effect of neurointensive care upon outcome following severe head injuries in childhood: A preliminary report. *Neuropediatrics*, *15*, 68–75.

Klonoff, H., Low, M. D., & Clark, C. (1977). Head injuries in children: A prospective five year follow-up. *Journal of Neurology, Neurosurgery and Psychiatry*, *40*, 1211–1219.

Kraus, J. F. (1987). Epidemiology of head injury. In P. R. Cooper (Ed.), *Head injury* (pp. 1–19). Baltimore: Williams & Wilkins.

Kraus, J. F., Fife, D., Cox, P., Ramstein, K., & Conroy, C. (1986). Incidence, severity and external causes of pediatric brain injury. *American Journal of Diseases of Children*, *140*, 687–693.

Kraus, J. F., Rock, A., & Hemyari, P. (1990). Brain injuries among infants, children, adolescents, and young adults. *American Journal of Diseases of Children*, *144*, 684–691.

Lanser, J. B., Jennekens-Schinkel, A., & Peters, A. C. (1988). Headache after closed head injury in children. *Headache*, *28*, 176–179.

Levin, H. S., Amparo, E., Eisenberg, H. M., Williams, D. H., High, W. A., McArdle, C. B., & Weiner, R. L. (1987). Magnetic resonance imaging and computerized tomography in relation to the neurobehavioral sequelae of mild and moderate head injuries. *Journal of Neurosurgery*, *66*, 706–713.

Levin, H. S., & Benton, A. L. (1986). Developmental and acquired dyscalculia in children. In I. Flehmig & I. Stern (Eds.), *Child development and learning behavior* (pp. 317–322). Stuttgart: Gustav Fisher.

Levin, H. S., Benton, A. L., & Grossman, R. G. (1982). *Neurobehavioral consequences of closed head injury*. New York: Oxford University Press.

Levin, H. S., & Eisenberg, H. M. (1979a). Neuropsychological impairment after closed head injury in children and adolescents. *Journal of Pediatric Psychology*, *4*, 389–402.

Levin, H. S., & Eisenberg, H. M. (1979b). Neuropsychological outcome of closed head injury in children and adolescents. *Child's Brain*, *5*, 281–292.

Levin, H. S., Eisenberg, H. M., Wigg, N. R., & Kobayashi, K. (1982). Memory and intellectual ability after head injury in children and adolescents. *Neurosurgery*, *11*, 668–673.

Levin, H. S., Ewing-Cobbs, L., & Fletcher, J. M. (1989). Neurobehavioral outcome of mild head injury in children. In H. S. Levin, H. M. Eisenberg, & A. L. Benton (Eds.), *Mild head injury* (pp. 189–213). New York: Oxford University Press.

Levin, H. S., Grafman, J., & Eisenberg, H. M. (1987). *Neurobehavioral Recovery from Head Injury*. New York: OxfordUniversity Press.

Levin, H. S., High, W. M., Ewing-Cobbs, L., Fletcher, J. M., Eisenberg, H. M., Miner, M., & Goldstein, F. C. (1988). Memory functioning during the first year after closed head injury in children and adolescents. *Neurosurgery*, *22*, 1043–1052.

Luerssen, T. G., Klauber, M., & Marshall, L. (1988). Outcome from head injury related to patient's age. *Journal of Neurosurgery*, *68*, 409–416.

Mahoney, W. J., D'Souza, B. J., Haller, J. A., Rogers, M. C., Epstein, M. H., & Freeman, J. M. (1983). Long-term outcome of children with severe head trauma and prolonged coma. *Pediatrics*, *77*, 756–762.

Mathews, J., Friman, P., Barone, V., Ross, L., & Christophersen, E. (1987). Decreasing dangerous infant behaviors through parent instruction. *Journal of Applied Behavior Analysis*, *20*, 165–169.

McGuire, T. L., & Sylvester, C. E. (1987). Neuropsychiatric evaluation and treatment of children with head injury. *Journal of Learning Disabilities*, *20*, 590–595.

Menkes, J. H., & Batzdorf, U. (1974). Post natal trauma and injuries by physical agents. In J. Menkes (Ed.), *Textbook of child neurology* (pp. 312–338). Philadelphia: Lea and Febiger.

Mickle, J. P. (1989). Acute head injuries in children. In *Conns Current Therapy* (pp. 841–844). Philadelphia: Saunders.

Parmelee, D. X., & O'Shanick, G. J. (1987). Neuropsychiatric interventions with head injured children and adolescents. *Brain Injury*, *1*, 41–47.

Prigatano, G. P., Fordyce, D. J., Zeiner, H. K., Roueche, J. R., Pepping, M., & Wood, B. C. (1984). Neuropsychological rehabilitation after closed head injury in young adults. *Journal of Neurology, Neurosurgery and Psychiatry*, *47*, 505–513.

Rivara, F. P., & Mueller, B. A. (1986). The epidemiology and prevention of pediatric head injury. *Journal of Head Trauma Rehabilitation*, *1*, 7–15.

Robinson, E. A., Eyberg, S., & Ross, A. W. (1980). Standardization of a behavior rating scale for conduct problem children. *Journal of Clinical Child Psychology*, *9*, 22–28.

Rutherford, W. H. (1989). Postconcussion symptoms: Relationship to acute neurological indices, individual differences and circumstances of injury. In H. S. Levin, H. M. Eisenberg, & P. L. Benton (Eds.), *Mild head injury* (pp. 217–227). New York: Oxford University Press.

Rutter, M., Chadwick, O., & Shaffer, D. (1984). Head injury. In M. Rutter (Ed.), *Developmental neuropsychiatry* (pp. 83–111). New York: Guilford Press.

Shaffer, D., Bijur, P., Chadwick, O., & Rutter, M. (1980). Head injury and later reading disability. *Journal of American Academy of Child Psychiatry*, *19*, 592–610.

Shapiro, K. (1987). Special considerations for the pediatric age group. In P. R. Cooper (Ed.), *Head injury* (pp. 367–389). Baltimore: Williams & Wilkins.

Shum, D., McFarland, K. A., & Bain, J. B. (1990). Validity of eight tests of attention: Comparison of normals and head injured samples. *The Clinical Neuropsychologist*, *4*, 151–162.

Slater, E. J., & Bassett, S. S. (1988). Adolescents with closed head injuries. *American Journal of Diseases of Children*, *142*, 1048–1051.

Snow, R. S., Zimmerman, R. D., Gandy, S. F., & Deck, M. D. (1986). Comparison of magnetic resonance imaging and computed tomography in the evaluation of head injury. *Neurosurgery*, *18*, 45–52.

Sparrow, S. S., Balla, D., & Chicchetti, D. (1984). *The Vineland Adaptive Behavior Scales*. Circle Pines, MN: American Guidance Service.

Speltz, M. L., Gonzales, N., Sulzbacher, S., & Quan, L. (1990). Assessment of injury risk in young children: A preliminary study of the Injury Behavior Checklist. *Journal of Pediatric Psychology*, *15*, 373–384.

Taylor, H. G. (1984). Early brain injury and cognitive development. In C. R. Almli & S. Finger (Eds.), *Early brain injury* (pp. 325–341). New York: Academic Press.

Teasdale, G., & Jennett, B. (1974). Assessment of coma and impaired consciousness: A practical scale. *Lancet*, *2*, 81–84.

Wilberger, J. F., Deeb, Z., & Rothfus, W. (1987). Magnetic resonance imaging in cases of severe head injury. *Neurosurgery*, *20*, 571–576.

Winogron, H. W., Knights, R. M., & Bawden, H. N. (1984). Neuropsychological deficits following head injury in children. *Journal of Clinical Neuropsychology*, *6*, 269–286.

Ylvisaker, M. (1986). Language and communication disorders following pediatric head injury. *Journal of Head Trauma Rehabilitation*, *1*, 48–56.

CHAPTER 3

Sequelae of *Haemophilus Influenzae* Meningitis: Implications for the Study of Brain Disease and Development

H. GERRY TAYLOR, CHRISTOPHER SCHATSCHNEIDER, and DEBORAH RICH

Early Brain Injuries

Consequences

Brain injuries that are present at birth or acquired in the first few years of life affect development in ways that are highly variable and poorly understood. Mental retardation is a common outcome for many of these children (Benton, 1962; Levin, Ewing-Cobbs, & Benton, 1987; Rutter, Graham, & Yule, 1970; St. James-Roberts, 1981). At the other end of the spectrum are individuals who make good developmental progress despite extensive early neuropathology (Smith & Sugar, 1975). What is remarkable about these latter cases—involving, for example, substantial tissue loss secondary to infantile hydrocephalus or removal of an entire hemisphere—is that injuries of similar severity in adulthood would have devastating effects. One observer has queried whether it might be advantageous "to have your brain lesion early" (Schneider, 1979, p. 557), and another if the brain is "really necessary" (Lewin, 1980, p. 1232).

Between these two extremes are children for whom the consequences of early brain injury are less certain, and the extent of "sparing" following early disease more problematic. Sequelae are often confounded with social and environmental factors, making it difficult to isolate the effects of the brain disease itself. There also may be uncertainty as to whether the initial disease permanently altered central nervous system (CNS) structure or function (Rutter, 1981; St. James-Roberts, 1981). Research linking childhood behavioral and learning problems to prenatal and perinatal complications exemplifies these dilemmas. Critiques of studies, such as that of Pasamanick and Knobloch (1961), indicate that social confounds were responsible, in large part, for the reported associations (Sameroff & Chandler, 1975). Prospective follow-up studies of premature children generally have failed to substantiate long-term sequelae unrelated to social factors (Kopp & Krakow, 1983). The fact that complications are more predictive of development immediately after birth than thereafter

(Greenberg & Crnic, 1988; Werner & Smith, 1982) raises doubts as to the permanence of CNS abnormalities.

On the other hand, it is clear that even definitive forms of early brain disease lead to diverse and highly variable outcomes, and that neurological abnormality need not be verifiable at the time of testing for sequelae to be present. Studies of children with histories of cerebral palsy, head injury, high lead burden, encephalitis, and other neurological disorders document problems in cognitive performance, learning, and behavior among nonretarded children with normal neurological examinations (Benton, 1962; Boll & Barth, 1981; Rutter, 1981; Taylor, 1984, 1987). Social factors or overt handicaps, such as seizures or hemiplegia, may contribute to the child's difficulties but do not account for them fully (Rutter, 1981; Seidel, Chadwick, & Rutter, 1975).

The primary research issue is not whether children with early brain damage experience sequelae, but how development is affected and the reasons for individual variations in outcome (Taylor, 1984). What, for example, accounts for variability in sparing across individuals? Is normal development, where observed, due to the absence of residual damage, neural reorganization, or behavioral compensation (St. James-Roberts, 1979)? What role do environmental and experiential factors play, and do these factors make more or less difference for the brain injured child as compared to other children?

Relevance

These issues are critical for both theory and practice. Follow-up studies of children with early brain disease are "experiments in nature" that have the potential to inform us about the role of the CNS in cognitive development. Correspondences between brain status and behavior offer insights as to which child behaviors are more reflective of biological as opposed to experiential variation, much in the same way that twin studies are useful in clarifying the influences of nature and nurture on IQ and other psychological traits (Plomin, 1989; Thompson, in press; Weinberg, 1989). Evaluations of brain injured children also can shed light on the joint contributions of biological and environmental factors to behavioral and learning disorders (Breslau, 1985; Rutter, 1981; Seidel et al., 1975; Taylor & Schatschneider, 1989). Showing that a particular behavioral characteristic is associated with the child's brain status is similar to demonstrating heritability. Evidence for brain relatedness does not imply that the characteristic is insensitive to environmental influences but only that biological variation accounts for some variability in function under existing environmental conditions (Angoff, 1988). In cases where there are selective consequences, behavioral dissociations brought about by brain injury are also revealing with respect to the structure of childhood abilities (e.g., Dennis, 1980).

The hypothesis that certain behavioral functions mirror brain status more directly than others has a long history. Based on observations of the differences between early and later occurring brain insults, Hebb (1942) postulated that there are two types of intelligence. According to Hebb's formulation, intellectual power (i.e., intelligence A) involves the ability to acquire new skills, solve novel problems by "synthesis and invention" (p. 257), and "develop a test ability in the absence of any previous relevant experience" (p. 287). Intellectual products (i.e., intelligence B), in contrast, encompass abilities acquired by virtue of experience. This distinction has been frequently recapitulated in the form of dichotomies between aptitude and achievement (Angoff, 1988; Hebb & Morton, 1944); in comparisons between fluid and crystallized intelligence and between learning processes and acquired knowledge (Cattell, 1963; Estes, 1981; Horn, 1968); and in the search for measures of "biological intelligence" (Reynolds, 1981; Vernon, 1981). A more recent case in point is Rourke's (1988) proposal that the neural mechanisms underlying novel learning should be considered separate from those that subserve assimilated skills. The cognitive profiles of children with early brain insults and the relationship of cognitive skills to academic and intellectual achievements have direct bearing on this hypothesis.

The effects of early brain disease provide clues regarding brain–behavior relationships in children, how these relationships change with age, and the potential of the young brain for reorganization of structure and function. Although there is little support for the view that young children are less vulnerable to brain injury than are adults (Fletcher, Levin, & Landry, 1984; St. James-Roberts, 1979), the consequences of early and later lesions are in many ways dissimilar. Unilateral lesions acquired before 1 year of age, for example, are not associated with verbal–performance IQ splits (Aram & Ekelman, 1986; Woods, 1980). Children who have localized disease within the first year of life are not necessarily free of impairment, but they are less likely to manifest the specific deficits that characterize adult lesions, such as prolonged aphasia (Alajouanine & Lhermitte, 1965; Aram, 1988; Byers & McLean, 1962; Dennis & Whitaker, 1976; Hecaen, 1976; Kohn & Dennis, 1974; Lenneberg, 1967; Satz & Bullard-Bates, 1981; Van Dongen & Loonen, 1977; Woods & Carey, 1979; Woods & Teuber, 1978).

Other unique features of early brain injury include the tendency for verbal abilities to develop at the expense of nonverbal skills (Lansdell, 1969; Teuber, 1975); diminished IQ (Boll & Barth, 1981; Taylor, 1984); greater sparing of elementary sensory compared to more complex functions (Laurence & Stein, 1978; Rudel, Teuber, & Twitchell, 1974); and for consequences to emerge long after the insult (Goldman & Lewis, 1978; Teuber & Rudel, 1962). The neurological, behavioral, and experiential processes responsible for these phenomena are the source of considerable theoretical speculation and controversy (Finger, LeVere,

Almli, & Stein, 1988; Kolb, 1989; St. James-Roberts, 1979; Taylor, 1984).

One of the practical advantages of investigating early brain injuries is a better appreciation of disease sequelae. This information is of value in establishing a prognosis and in deciding on the importance of preventive efforts. Identification of variables that place children at greatest risk for sequelae is also clinically relevant. If risks are known, the clinician can focus resources where they are most needed and increase the chances of early recognition of any developmental problems. Environmental conditions or child traits associated with a lower risk for sequelae may also reveal "protective" factors (Masten & Garmezy, 1985).

Further practical benefits are the treatment implications of research findings. Discovery of correlates of positive outcomes may suggest ways to minimize potentially adverse effects. If cognitive limitations are understood, recommendations can be made for special help or accommodation (Rourke, Fisk, & Strang, 1986; Ylvisaker, 1985). Appreciation of post-injury changes in functioning are also relevant in giving parents and teachers advice regarding the child's ability to meet age-appropriate expectations (Crothers & Lord, 1938; Fuld & Fisher, 1977).

Aims

The major purpose of this chapter is to describe a research program initiated several years ago to investigate the school-age consequences of *Haemophilus influenzae* type b (Hib) meningitis. There were several reasons why this particular disease was chosen for study. To begin with, Hib meningitis represents a relatively common and potentially lethal form of postnatal brain disease that is contracted by previously normal children, and well within the first 5 years of life. When the present research program was initiated, immunizations had not been developed; the immunizations currently available are not yet fully effective. Popular opinion, moreover, is that a high percentage of children who have recovered from Hib meningitis exhibit specific developmental disabilities. Hib meningitis was thus an appropriate disease for investigation of more subtle or isolated forms of sequelae.

Despite the general sense of a relatively poor prognosis, much of the existing literature was methodologically flawed. The "common wisdom" regarding sequelae appeared to be based on studies involving potentially biased samples, inadequate control groups, and lack of comprehensive or standardized outcome measures. The pilot study for the current research program was a response to the need for more methodologically sound research on postmeningitis developmental outcomes. A cohort of children who had survived this disease had been actively followed by Dr. Richard Michaels at the Children's Hospital of Pittsburgh and was available for recruitment.

The research that was carried out with this patient sample, together with the National Institutes of Health–supported project to which it led, had two major objectives. The first goal was to clarify the consequences of Hib meningitis. The second was to explore medical and social risks for adverse outcomes. Our primary aims in this chapter are to describe the broader framework for the study, review rationale and procedures, highlight major methodological issues, and consider the significance of preliminary findings and their implications for future work in this area.

The first section of this chapter provides an overview of the consequences of early brain injury and of the factors that are predictive of outcome. This existing knowledge base helped to shape our hypotheses and to influence selection of outcome measures and predictor variables. The second section reviews the literature on Hib meningitis. The present research program is described in the third section. Emphasis in this section is on the conceptual framework guiding this work and the methodology employed to address our research questions. Because findings are as yet preliminary and data analysis incomplete, results to date are only briefly summarized to illustrate the extent to which hypotheses have been confirmed and to underscore methodological and conceptual issues. The final section focuses on the significance of these preliminary findings, methodological limitations, and implications for future research.

Important Variables

Measures of Outcome

As noted earlier, the effects of early brain disease range widely. Whereas some children sustain no apparent consequences, others are frankly retarded or manifest any number of more specific disabilities. IQ is generally depressed in groups of children with definitive forms of brain injury, even discounting those with mental retardation. In fact, omnibus IQ measures such as the Wechsler Intelligence Scales for Children–Revised, or WISC-R (Wechsler, 1974), have proved to be highly sensitive to differences between brain injured and control groups (Boll & Barth, 1981; Reitan, 1974; Rutter, 1981). Depending on age at injury and lesion location, verbal abilities can be as much or more affected than nonverbal skills (Fletcher et al., 1984). More typically, however, Performance IQ is reduced relative to Verbal IQ (Boll & Barth, 1981; Dennis et al., 1981; Fletcher & Copeland, 1988; Fletcher & Levin, 1988; Levin et al., 1987; Rutter, 1981; Taylor, Michaels, Mazur, Bauer, & Liden, 1984). The opportunity to compare Verbal and Performance IQ makes the WISC-R an attractive choice for intellectual assessment.

In addition to its effects on IQ, brain disease can lead to any number of sequelae. Consequences vary widely with no characteristic pattern. It is therefore mandatory to evaluate a wide range of specific cognitive functions (Boll & Barth, 1981; Rourke, Bakker, Fisk, & Strang, 1983; Taylor & Fletcher, 1990). Functional areas most likely to be affected in nonretarded children are visuomotor and perceptual–organizational skills, psychomotor speed, attention, learning and memory, and abstract reasoning (Bawden, Knights, & Winogron, 1985; Benton, 1962; Birch & Bortner, 1967; Fletcher & Copeland, 1988; Levin et al., 1987; Lord, 1937; Taylor, 1959; Taylor, 1987). In the language domain, comprehension of syntax, lexical retrieval, and fluency may be especially vulnerable (Aram, 1988; Dennis, Hendrick, Hoffman, & Humphreys, 1987; Ewing-Cobbs, Levin, Eisenberg, & Fletcher, 1987). An additional requirement is to examine individual outcomes rather than to focus solely on comparison of group means. Study of the effects of brain disease on individuals is useful in identifying risks for sequelae, in gauging the real-life consequences of the disease (e.g., percentage of children requiring special education), and in determining the representativeness of group differences.

In a study that illustrates this approach to assessment, Taylor Albo, Phebus, Sachs, and Bierl (1987) administered a large battery of tests to children who had received irradiation for treatment of acute lymphocytic leukemia (ALL). They also obtained ratings and other information on behavior and school performance from each child's parents and teacher. The effect of treatment for ALL was assessed by means of paired comparisons of these children to their siblings. Results indicated that group differences were more pronounced on some tasks than on others. Consistent with the literature cited, the ALL group seemed to have most difficulty relative to their siblings on tasks of novel learning or problem solving, visual-motor skill, psychomotor speed, memory, and attentional control. Examination of the distribution of WISC-R Full Scale IQs (see Figure 3.1) suggested that prophylactic irradiation for ALL results in a downward shift relative to siblings in the entire distribution of scores. Group differences, in other words, were not due to a few extreme cases. The latter information, which was not available in comparison of group means, indicates that the consequences of ALL treatment might be best conceptualized as a slight lowering of IQ across a large proportion of the survivors.

Problems in academic achievement and school performance are often reported and are not necessarily accounted for by IQ. In spite of the generally average IQs of the ALL children studied by Taylor, Albo, et al. (1987), their academic achievement and school performance were significantly below those of the sibling controls. These differences had clear implications for individual children: almost three times as many of the ALL children were receiving special educational assistance, and more than twice as many had been retained at least one grade in school. Similarly, Aram and Ekelman (1988) found that children with early

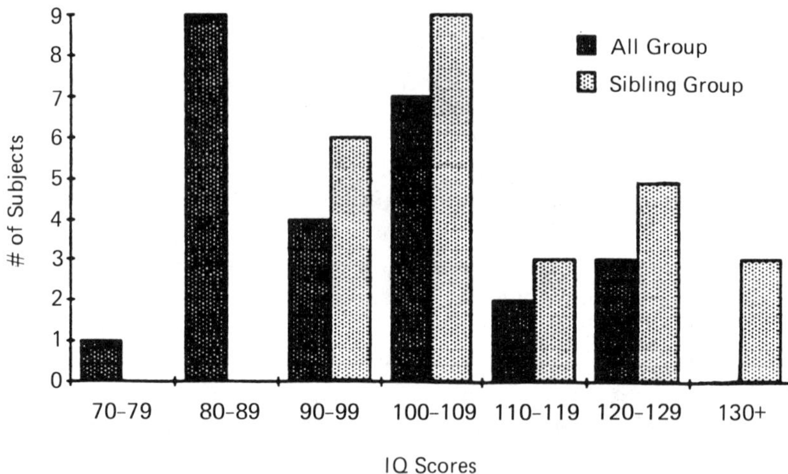

Fig. 3.1. Distribution of Full Scale IQ scores (WISC-R) in the ALL and sibling groups. From "Postirradiation Treatment Outcomes for Children with Acute Lymphocytic Leukemia: Clarification of Risks" by H. Taylor, V. Albo, C. Phoebus, B. Sachs, and P. Bierl, 1987, *Journal of Pediatric Psychology*, *12*, p. 401. Copyright 1987 by Plenum Publishing Corporation. Reprinted by permission.

unilateral lesions, all of whom had normal IQs, performed more poorly than controls on tests of academic achievement. Klein, Hack, and Breslau (1989) observed that children born at very low birth weight (i.e., <1500 grams) had deficiencies in math relative to full-term children, even when comparison was restricted to children with IQs of 85 and greater. Further, Seidel et al. (1975) documented poor reading achievement in a heterogeneous sample of brain injured children which was not accounted for by either limited IQ or associated physical handicaps.

Behavioral problems constitute another ecologically meaningful correlate of brain injury. Although no one behavioral pattern is characteristic, clinical descriptions emphasize emotional instability, inconsistency, unmanageability, and poor impulse control (e.g., Benton, 1962; Crothers & Lord, 1938). Using standardized parent behavioral ratings, Thompson, Kronenberger, Johnson, and Whiting (1989) found that 52% of a sample of children with myelodysplasia were judged to have behavioral or social difficulties. Kindlon, Sollee, and Yando (1988) report a similar incidence of behavior problems in a group of children with documented brain disease (based on the presence of a neurological disorder or laboratory evidence of neuropathology). Data from numerous investigations of brain injured children indicate a raised incidence of psychiatric disturbance that cannot be explained in terms of low IQ, chronic illness, or physical handicaps (Breslau, 1985, 1990; Breslau, Klein, & Allen, 1988; Breslau & Marshall, 1985; Rutter, 1977, 1981).

Brown, Chadwick, Shaffer, Rutter, and Traub (1981) offer further support for the need to evaluate postinsult changes in behavior. These researchers found that about half of a sample of children who had sustained severe head trauma developed psychiatric disorders postinjury that were not apparent prior to the trauma. This rate of new disorders was more than three times the rate observed in a group of orthopedically injured controls. Long-term effects on behavior and adaptive abilities in head injured children also have been documented by Perrott, Taylor, and Montes (1991), and Fletcher, Ewing-Cobbs, Miner, Levin, and Eisenberg (1990). The lack of close correspondence between cognitive and behavioral outcomes in these and other studies argues for the need to assess both types of sequelae.

These findings argue for comprehensive evaluations of outcomes following early brain insults. Thorough assessment entails tests of general intelligence, together with procedures for evaluating a number of more specific neurocognitive functions. These latter functions include language competencies, motor and somatosensory skills, perceptual-motor and constructional abilities, learning and memory, attention and psychomotor efficiency, and abstract reasoning (Taylor & Fletcher, 1990). Criteria to consider in selecting tests are (1) satisfaction of the usual standards for psychometric adequacy; (2) measurement of separable, unidimensional skills as well as integrative abilities; (3) availability of age-related norms and sensitivity to developmental differences; (4) validity in discriminating brain injured children from normal children; and (5) validity in predicting ecologically meaningful aspects of child development, such as learning, behavior, and adaptive abilities (Rourke, Fisk, & Strang, 1986; Taylor, 1988; Taylor & Fletcher, 1990; Taylor & Schatschneider, 1990). Appraisal of academic achievement, school performance, behavior, social skills, and other adaptive characteristics is also warranted.

Predictors

The understanding of how brain injuries influence behavior and the appreciation of disease effects on individuals also require examination of the correlates, or predictors, of outcome. As stated by St. James-Roberts, the purpose of research in this area "is not to isolate direct effects of CNS insult so much as to question whether early insults limit the function so identified to a significant degree relative to other exigencies" (1979, p. 300). The complexity of these other influences is illustrated by the long list of factors that Rutter (1977, 1981) suggested for consideration as contributors to postinsult psychiatric disturbance. Included in this list are disease severity; the child's premorbid adjustment; postinjury medical complications or treatments; changes in personality following the insult, even if temporary; prevailing social/familial circumstances; the reaction of the child and others to events surrounding the disease; and the child's ability to meet postinjury behavioral, cognitive, or academic demands. Several of these variables are discussed next.

Nature of Insult

One critical determinant of outcome is the nature and extent of brain injury. Children with diffuse bilateral insults do more poorly, in general, than children with focal damage. Evidence in this regard comes from findings indicating that (1) bilateral disease has more significant consequences than unilateral disease (Rutter et al., 1970; Satz, 1987); (2) size of lesion is correlated with intelligence in acquired hemiplegics (Banich, Levine, Kim, & Huttenlocher, 1990); (3) more destructive grades of intracerebral hemorrhage in the neonate are associated with poorer developmental outcomes (Fletcher et al., 1984); and (4) indices of head injury severity (e.g., duration of coma, period of posttraumatic amnesia, and degree of neurological abnormalities accompanying the trauma) are predictive of posttraumatic cognitive and behavioral status (Fletcher & Levin, 1988).

Other neuropathological determinants of outcome are lesion locus, type of pathology, presence of seizures or other neurological complications, and rate of progression of the lesion (Birch, 1981, Broman, Nichols, & Kennedy, 1975; Drillien, Thomson, & Burgoyne, 1980; Hack & Breslau, 1986; Rourke et al., 1986; Rutter, 1981; Van Dongen & Loonen, 1977; Vohr & Coll, 1985; Wiener Rider, Oppel, Fischer, & Harper, 1965). Investigations of the effects of locus of lesion suggest that left-hemisphere disease, even in the young brain, predisposes the child to higher level linguistic impairment (Aram, 1988; Dennis & Whitaker, 1976). Early right-hemisphere disease, in contrast, can lead to perceptual deficits with a relative sparing of language functions (Kohn & Dennis, 1974; Woods, 1980). Other findings suggest that subcortical disease may have more adverse consequences than cortical injuries (Aram & Ekelman, 1986, 1988; Rutter, 1981). Nor surprisingly, children whose disease is accompanied by definitive neurological symptoms are at greater risk for sequelae than children without such symptoms (Hack & Breslau, 1986; Klein, Feigin, & McCracken, 1986; Vohr & Coll, 1985).

Age at Insult

Contrary to the notion of early neural plasticity, numerous findings suggest that consequences may be more adverse the earlier the age at insult (Davidson, Willoughby, O'Luam, Swisher, & Benjamins, 1978; Ewing-Cobbs, Levin, Eisenberg, & Fletcher, 1987; Fletcher & Copeland, 1988; Levin, Eisenberg, Wiig, & Kobayashi, 1982; Taylor et al., 1984). Recovery from aphasia following left-hemisphere insult is nonetheless more rapid and complete in younger children, and laterality of dysfunction (language versus nonlanguage) is less prominent for early than for later unilateral lesions (Annett, 1973; Lansdell, 1969; Teuber, 1975; Vargha-Khadem, Isaacs, Papaleloudi, Polkey, & Wilson, in press; Vargha-Khadem, O'Gorman, & Watters, 1985; Woods, 1980; Woods & Carey, 1979).

Although there is no clear line of demarcation between early and later insults, most research in this area distinguishes later postnatal lesions (i.e., after age 5) from injuries occurring prior to that time. A distinction is also made between prenatal or early postnatal insults (i.e., up to age 1 or 2) and those occurring in the preschool years (Aram & Ekelman, 1986; Lansdell, 1969; Rasmussen & Milner, 1977; Teuber, 1975; Vargha-Khadem et al., 1985). Satz's (1987) review of the evidence led him to conclude that interhemispheric reorganization of both speech and handedness is most likely when insults occur before 1 year of age. According to Satz, left-hemisphere insults from age 1 to 6 years result in less complete shifts, whereas damage sustained after this age is less commonly associated with interhemispheric shifts in either speech dominance or handedness.

Age at Testing and Time Postinsult

Obstacles that researchers face in comparing the effects of lesions occurring at different ages are confounds involving age at insult, age at testing, and time postinsult (St. James-Roberts, 1981; Vargha-Khadem et al., 1985; Witelson, 1987). Recognition of these confounds is important for several reasons. First, the initial effect of the injury may be especially pronounced due to "diaschisis," or the generalized depression of neural function related to edema, biochemical disruptions, or neuronal degeneration. "Emergence trauma," or concurrent illness or hospitalization, may have a similar impact (St. James-Roberts, 1981). To the extent that these effects dissipate over time, sequelae may appear to be greater in children with later occurring injuries, but only because postinjury follow-up periods are shorter than in children with early lesions. These transitory depressions of function also may make it difficult to predict longer term effects immediately postinjury. Second, a longer period of follow-up may result in progressive gains or losses in ability over time. Such changes further obscure the influence of age at insult. Finally, comparison of outcomes at widely different ages may have little meaning. Sequelae may themselves be age related, and scores from even structurally similar test procedures may be incomparable (Taylor & Fletcher, in press). Proper investigation of age as it relates to sparing demands factorial variation in each of these variables, usually made unfeasible by real-world constraints.

Study of the effects of age at testing on outcome is nevertheless of importance for its own sake, especially because it is often possible to restrict age at injury within reasonably narrow limits. Animal studies described by Goldman and her colleagues (Goldman, 1974; Goldman & Lewis, 1978) suggest that some neural structures are "prefunctional." Early damage to these areas fails to have immediate effects but will limit subsequent development. A similar process has been proposed for human development. Increasing localization of function and neural "commitment" are postulated to arise from the working of wider neural systems in the young brain. Early damage will therefore set greater limits on development than injury sustained later in life (Hebb, 1942; Piercy, 1964; Russell, 1948; Vygotsky, 1962).

Observations from clinical follow-up of brain damaged children have been consistent with this "cumulative deficit" model. Myer and Byers, for example, described intellectual deterioration over time in children with measles encephalitis, which they ascribed to an "inability to acquire new knowledge and adaptations" (1952, p. 555). More recent confirmation is provided by cross-sectional studies carried out by Banich et al. (1990), Dennis et al. (1987), Fletcher et al. (1990), and Wills, Holmbeck, Dillon, and McLone (1990), as well as by longitudinal findings reported by Breslau and Marshall (1985) and Fletcher, Levin, and Landry (1984). In each case, failure to develop according to age expectations can be accounted for in terms of either a retarded rate of learning or increasing demands for those higher order skills most compromised by the insult. Changes in motivation or environmental supports (e.g., declining effort or coping, lowered self-esteem, increased sensitivity to problems, and less assistance or accommodation) also bear consideration.

Other evidence, however, fails to indicate a worsening of sequelae with age at testing or time postinsult. Recovery in IQ continues for long periods post–head injury (Levin et al., 1987). Increments in IQ with age also have been reported in children with early hydrocephalus and hemispherectomy (St. James-Roberts, 1981). Dependencies of postinsult changes on the assessment measure, IQ level, premorbid behavior, and the child's experiences before and after brain injury may help to explain these apparent disparities (Chadwick, Rutter, Brown, Shaffer, & Traub, 1981; Kolb, 1989; Rutter, 1977, 1981; St. James-Roberts, 1979).

Gender

Because psychiatric disturbances and developmental disabilities are more prevalent among males than females (Cullinan, Epstein, & Lloyd, 1981; Kopp, 1983; Nichols & Chen, 1981; Rutter, 1982), a similar sex difference might be anticipated in investigating outcomes following early brain injury. Several studies of children with known or suspected histories of early brain insult do, in fact, report a greater incidence of behavior problems in males than in females (Klonoff & Low, 1974; Parkinson, Wallis, & Harvey, 1981; Streissguth, Barr, Sampson, Darby, & Martin, 1989). In one of the best controlled studies to date, Breslau et al. (1988) compared 9-year-old children born at very low birth weight to full-term controls on standardized ratings of behavior and social competence. Boys exhibited more behavior problems and lower social competence compared to sex-matched controls, but this was not the case in corresponding comparisons of females. The authors interpreted their findings with reference to sex-related differences in disease severity, in response to illness, or in the manner in which behavioral disturbance is manifested in the two sexes at various ages. Other studies report a trend in the opposite direction, with academic and cognitive disturbance secondary to early neurological disorder being more apparent in females than in males (Waber, Urion, & Tarbell, 1990). Further research is needed to investigate reasons for this disparity, but it is clear that potential sex differences warrant inclusion of this variable in investigation of disease consequences.

Social/Environmental Factors

Like gender, social variables such as socioeconomic status (SES), life events, and the home environment have an undisputed relationship to cognitive, behavioral, and academic development (Bradley, Caldwell, & Rock, 1989; Garmezy, Masten, & Tellegen, 1984; Sines, 1987). The strong associations of social factors and early experiences to outcomes following early brain insults are well documented and are perhaps the most consistently reported and unequivocal findings in the literature (Cohen, 1986; Davie, Butler, & Goldstein, 1972; Escalona, 1982; Hack & Breslau, 1986; Kolb, 1989; Rutter, 1981; Sameroff & Chandler, 1975; Thompson et al., 1989; Wallander, Varni, Babani, Banis, & Wilcox, 1989; Werner & Smith, 1982).

A more controversial issue is whether these factors have more influence on brain injured children relative to non–brain injured children, or whether the brain injured child is at "double hazard" (Escalona, 1982). At the center of this controversy is the meaning of a true interaction effect. The fact that the effects of conditions that place children at biological risk (e.g., prematurity) are amplified in those from more socially disadvantaged homes is not evidence of interaction. Augmentation of the effects of disease would occur if social risks merely added to adverse outcomes. What is required for demonstration of an interaction effect is that social conditions or learning history has a *greater or lesser* effect on children with brain disease than on other children.

Evidence in this regard is largely negative. In their studies of children with cerebral palsy, epilepsy, and head injuries, Rutter and his associates (Rutter, 1977) found that increased rates of behavioral distrubance were associated with both brain disease and social disadvantage, but that the two effects were additive rather than interactive. As illustrated in Figure 3.2, the impact of psychosocial disadvantage was to increase the rate of behavioral disturbance by about the same amount in both the brain injured and control groups.

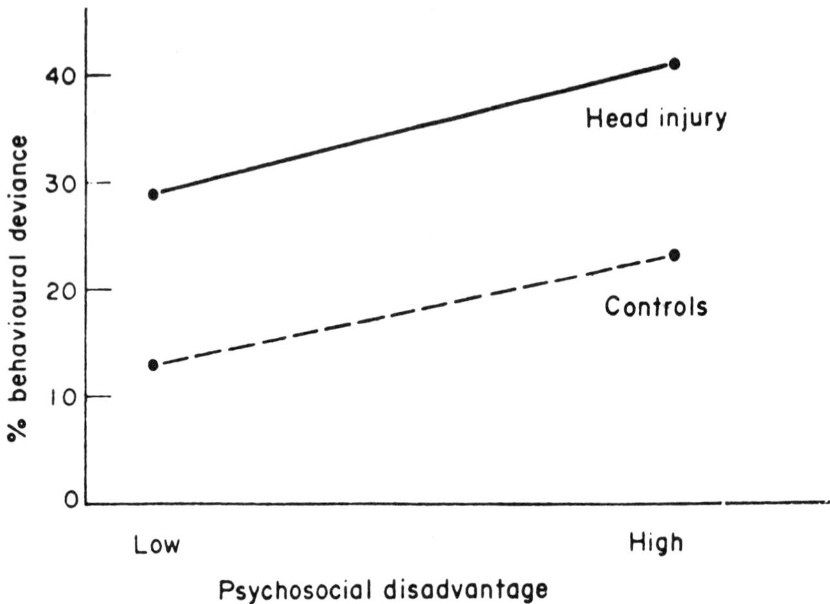

Fig. 3.2. Impact of psychosocial disadvantage on behavioral deviance. From "Brain Damage Syndromes in Children: Concepts and Findings" by M. Rutter, 1977, *Journal of Child Psychology and Psychiatry*, *18*, p. 10. Copyright 1977 by Pergamon, Press Plc. Reprinted by permission.

Breslau (1990) also failed to find social factors to be of any greater relevance to behavior in children with brain-related conditions (e.g., cerebral palsy, myelodysplasia, or multiple handicaps) than in normal controls. In her study, group membership predicted both depressive symptoms and inattention. Depressive symptoms, but not inattention, also were predicted by a measure of the family environment. However, there was no support for the hypothesis that children with brain insults are more vulnerable to nonoptimal family environments. In fact, Breslau found that the family environment was more predictive of inattention in control children than in those with brain injuries. One possibility raised by Breslau to explain this result is that brain injuries may tend to "insulate" the child from psychosocial influences.

An alternative to the double hazard hypothesis is the idea that social advantage may facilitate compensatory processes. According to this view, social advantage may be more essential for optimal development in brain injured children than in normal children. As in the case of the double hazard model, differences between brain damaged and normal children will tend to be greater at lower levels of social advantage. The reason for this, however, is not the potentiating influence of social disadvantage but the compensatory effects of social advantages. In essence, the compensation hypothesis emphasizes factors that mitigate against the otherwise untoward effects of brain disease—just as "protective" or resistance factors have been proposed to account for the failure of some high-risk individuals to develop psychopathology (Masten & Garmezy, 1985).

A consistent finding in follow-up of premature infants is that positive social factors ameliorate initial depressions in development related to prenatal and perinatal complications (Sameroff & Chandler, 1975; Vohr & Garcia-Coll, 1988). One example of how protective factors might be at work is provided by Siegel (1981), who found that infants who were classified incorrectly as at risk based on a 12 month assessment—that is, the false positives—were rated as having more stimulating home environments than the true positive cases.

A second illustration is given in research by Crnic and associates (Crnic, Ragozin, Greenberg, Robinson, & Basham, 1983; Greenberg & Crnic, 1988). These investigators found differences between preterm and term infants across a wide range of developmental measures during the first year of life. By 2 years of age, however, these same groups differed only in motor development. Of special relevance to this discussion is the fact that development at 2 years was more strongly related to earlier maternal behavior and the home environment in the preterm group than in full-term controls. Furthermore, the mothers of preterm infants who were at greater biological risk reported more positive feelings about their children at 1 month of age than did mothers of the preterm infants at lesser risk. The latter advantage, in turn, was related to more positive infant behaviors at 8 months. Greenberg and Crnic interpret their results with reference to "the transactional notion of compensatory or self-righting mechanisms within the caregiving context" (1988, p. 567).

The major limitation of this research with respect to the hypothesis of a brain–environment interaction is the questionable nature of the CNS insults involved (St. James-Roberts, 1979). A stronger case for interaction requires direct test of these effects in groups with more clear-cut brain injuries. Few studies have been designed for proper tests of interaction effects. It also is recognized that interactions, to the extent that they do exist, may apply only within a given range of disease severity or to certain types of outcomes; and that Breslau's (1990) insulation hypothesis has as much support as the double hazard or compensatory hypothesis.

Hib Meningitis

Background

Hib meningitis is the most common form of bacterial infection of the meningeal tissues, which surround the brain and spinal cord. Neuropathological studies indicate that this disease in accompanied by vascular inflammation and vessel occlusion throughout the CNS, cerebral edema, hydrocephalus, and subdural effusions (Headings & Glasgow, 1977; Herson & Todd, 1977; Klein et al., 1986; Sell, 1983; Swartz, 1984; Thomas & Hopkins, 1972). Serious sequelae stem primarily from ischemia resulting from altered cerebral blood flow, and from direct compression and herniation of the brain (Klein et al., 1986). In view of radiological evidence of infarction and ventricular enlargement (Snyder, Stovring, Cushing, Davis, & Hardy, 1981), brian insult is likely diffuse with areas of localized neuronal loss.

The annual incidence of Hib meningitis is 30 to 70/100,000 children under 5 years of age (Klein et al., 1986; Michaels & Schultz, 1973; Sell, 1983; Swaiman & Wright, 1982). In certain ethnic groups, such as Navajo Indians and Alaskan Yupik Eskimos, the incidence of this disease is many times greater (Coulehan et al., 1976; Fraser, 1982). Although Hib meningitis can be contracted by persons of any age, figures provided by Klein et al. (1986) suggest that 99% of the cases occur prior to age 5 years. Peak occurrence (77% of cases) is between 3 and 12 months of age. Genetic mechanisms have been proposed to account for ethnic differences. Sociodemographic and environmental factors, such as family size and proximity, also have been implicated in disease transmission (Fraser, 1982; Klein et al., 1986; Michaels & Schultz, 1973).

Presenting clinical symptoms include fever, irritability, lethargy, and vomiting (Klein et al., 1986; Swaiman & Wright, 1982). A stiff neck, seizures, bulging fontanel, and depressed consciousness may also signal the disease but may be more or less detectable depending on the child's age and disease state. Because initial symptoms are subjective and may be found in association with less serious forms of febrile illnesses, the diagnosis is confirmed by growth of the bacterium in cultures taken by lumber puncture from the cerebrospinal fluid (CSF).

A number of neurological complications in addition to seizures may arise over the course of the illness. These include cranial nerve deficits such as facial palsy; hemiparesis or quadriparesis; coma; blindness or visual field defects; sensorineural hearing loss; ataxia; cranial tomography (CT) findings suggestive of hydrocephalus, edema, large subdural effusions, or cortical atrophy; and abnormal electroencephalograms (EEGs). The disease also can result in shock, apnea, papilledema, and cardiopulmonary arrest (Dodge & Swartz, 1965; Klein et al., 1986; Lebel et al., 1988). Hearing loss, one of the most common disease complications, results from eighth nerve damage sustained when infection or inflammatory processes spread along the auditory canal and cochlear aqueduct (Sell, 1983).

The conventional treatment for Hib meningitis is to place the child on a 10 day course of ampicillin. Chloramphenicol is given initially in combination with ampicillin; it is withdrawn once it has been established that the bacteria are not ampicillin-resistant. Alternative antibiotic therapies, such as chloramphenicol, cefuroxime, and ceftriaxone, may be useful with resistant strains of bacteria (Klein et al., 1986; Schaad et al., 1990). Fluids are managed carefully and frequent neurological examinations and laboratory assays are conducted during hospitalization. EEGs and CT scans are performed electively to investigate possible complications. Recently developed immunizations have been shown to be effective in reducing disease incidence (Eskola et al., 1987). Methods of reducing risks of sequelae in children who have contracted Hib meningitis are also under study (Lebel et al., 1988).

Sequelae

Mortality from Hib meningitis exceeded 90% prior to the development of antibiotics (Kresky, Buchbinder, & Greenberg, 1962). Death rates have decreased substantially over the last 40 to 50 years and are now well below 10% (Klein et al., 1986). Nevertheless, there has been serious concern with regard to morbidity, which some investigators have suggested may involve as many as half of the survivors (Klein et al., 1986). Neurological sequelae have been found in up to one-third of the children in some samples (Kresky et al., 1962; Sell, Merrill, Doyne, & Zimsky, 1972; Sproles, Azerrad, Williamson, & Merrill, 1969). According to the existing research, these sequelae consist of permanent sensorineural hearing impairment in 0% to 30% of the children who recover, with a 10% rate believed to be generally representative (Dodge et al., 1984; Sell, 1983). Estimates of frank mental retardation (IQ < 70) range from 2% to 17% (Feigin et al., 1976; Ferry, Culbertson, Cooper, Sitton, & Sell, 1982; Klein et al., 1986; Lindberg, Rosenhall, Nylen, & Ringner, 1977; Sell, 1983; Sproles et al., 1969). Other residual neurological disorders are seizures in up to 30% of the cases (Dodge & Swartz, 1965; Feigin et al., 1976; Ferry et al., 1982; Jadavji, Biggar, Gold, & Prober, 1986; Sell, 1983), hemiparesis or other motor defect in 2% to 7% (Dodge & Swartz, 1965; Feigin et al., 1976; Jadavji et al., 1986; Sell, 1983), and visual impairment in 0% to 4% (Jadavji et al., 1986; Sell, 1983).

Delays in speech and language development, subnormal IQ and other cognitive deficits, school problems, and behavioral disturbances also have been cited (Feigin et al., 1976; Jadavji et al., 1986; Kresky et al., 1962; Lindberg et al., 1977; Sell, 1983; Sell, Merrill et al., 1972; Sproles et al., 1969; Wright & Jimmerson, 1971). Although the incidence of these particular problems is often unspecified, Sproles et al. reported that 28% of the survivors they assessed had "definite handicaps" involving "mild depression in the intelligence quotient, poor school performance, abnormality of electroencephalogram, hearing loss, speech deficit, minimal brain dysfunction, and behavioral problems" (1969, p. 786). Kresky et al. (1962) observed a 20% rate of poor school performance not explained by IQ, and Sell, Merrill, et al. (1972) observed isolated school failure in 14% of their sample. In one of the more systematic studies of developmental sequelae, Sell, Webb, Pate, and Doyne (1972) compared a group of 21 children who had recovered from Hib meningitis to 21 near-age siblings. The mean WISC IQ of the postmeningitis group was significantly lower than that of the siblings (86 vs. 97). Furthermore, whereas no postmeningitis child outperformed his or her sibling by 15 or more IQ points, siblings outscored postmeningitis children by this amount in 29% of the pairs.

Predictors

Previous research suggests that several disease-related variables may be useful in predicting outcomes following Hib meningitis. Lindberg et al. (1977) found subdural effusions and coma to be more common in survivors with neurological, intellectual, or behavioral impairments than in those without evidence of sequelae. Herson and Todd (1977) and Alon, Naveh, Gardos, and Friedman (1979) concluded that variables predictive of death or neurological sequelae were coma, seizures, hypothermia, shock, younger age at illness, longer pretreatment symptom duration, low hemoglobin, low CSF white cell count, and low CSF glucose concentration. According to Klein et al. (1986), seizures are prognostic of later neurological abnormalities only if they are focal or occur later in illness. Disease factors that have been associated with hearing loss and speech impairment include seizures prior to admission, in-hospital fever duration, duration of symptoms prior to treatment, concentrations of pretreatment bacterial antigen, and low CSF glucose—whether considered alone or as a ratio of blood glucose (Borkowski, Goldgar, Gorga, Brookhouser, & Worthington, 1985; Feldman et al., 1982; Kaplan, Catlin, Weaver, & Feigin, 1984; Lebel et al., 1988). Deficiencies in postmeningitis cognitive status have been related to younger age at illness, longer fever duration, and focal neurological findings during the acute phase of illness (Emmett, Jeffery, Chandler, & Dugdale, 1980; Klein et al., 1986). Finally, although randomized clinical trials have failed to reveal dependencies of outcome on antibiotic therapy (Feigin et al., 1976; Sell, 1983), Schaad et al. (1990) found ceftriaxone superior to cefuroxime in terms of bacteriocidal action and minimization of hearing loss.

Critique

Unfortunately, methodological limitations prevent one from drawing any firm conclusions from most of the research summarized here. Studies in this area rarely have included control groups. Without proper controls, one cannot be certain if deficiencies in cognitive, learning, or behavioral functions represent disease effects or are variations of normal development. Associations of the disease with sociodemographic factors makes this an especially pressing concern (Fraser, 1982). Furthermore, whereas at least two studies have found that postmeningitis children perform more poorly than controls on IQ tests (Sell, Webb, et al., 1972; Wright & Jimmerson, 1971), several others have failed to show lowered IQ relative to siblings (Emmett et al., 1980; Klein et al., 1986; Tejani, Dobias, & Sambursky, 1982). Doubts may be raised, therefore, as to the severity of disease consequences.

The lack of comprehensive or formalized assessment procedures has been another major shortcoming of research in this area. Problems in behavior or school performance frequently have been based on clinical impressions, interview, or examination of school records. Formal assessment, using age-normed and standardized instruments, has been largely limited to IQ testing. Speech and language development and academic skills have been evaluated objectively in a few instances (e.g., Feigin et al., 1976; Tejani et al., 1982). Prior to the present research program, however, no study of postmeningitis outcomes had utilized neuropsychological assessment methods. Without more thorough evaluations, it is difficult to know the full range of consequences and whether some types of outcomes may be more affected than others. The study of disease factors that are predictive of sequelae also would be fostered by more systematic evaluation of outcomes.

A third problem concerns the sampling techniques used in previous studies of postmeningitis outcomes. Many investigations have used rigorous procedures for sample recruitment, with patients recruited either prospectively or from retrospective review of all children treated within a given time frame. Other reports concerning sampling procedures have been vague, and sample representativeness is therefore suspect. One way to determine the representativeness of findings would be to recruit subjects from multiple hospital sites, employing consistent procedures, and then to compare findings across sites. Recruitment from multiple sites additionally would address the issue of limited sample sizes. Small samples restrict statistical power for detection of relationships between disease parameters and outcomes. Larger samples would be useful in examining associations between multiple risk factors and developmental outcomes and in determining the significance of low-incidence events (e.g., neurological complications during the acute phase of the illness). Previous investigations have tended to base risk estimates on bivariate correlations between illness variables and outcomes and on clinical judgment as to how factors should be weighted to establish a composite risk score (Herson & Todd, 1977; Wright, 1978). Multiple regression techniques, which require larger samples, would be preferable for a more empirically based study of disease-related risks.

A final limitation is that past work in this area has not considered variables that may serve to moderate the effects of disease on development. Although age at illness has received some attention as a disease variable, factors such as age at testing, sex, and social/environmental condition have been ignored. Although some sequelae may be present for all age, sex, and social groups, other consequences may be specific to, or at least more marked in, select subgroups of children. Failure to include subject factors in examining disease effects has two disadvantages. First, disease effects may be so subtle as to be obscured unless such factors are taken into account. Second, as discussed earlier in this chapter, dependencies of disease consequences on these factors would shed light on the ways in which early brain insults affect development.

The Present Research Program

Rationale and Hypotheses

The intent of the present research program was to investigate the childhood consequences of Hib meningitis using more rigorous methodology than employed in previous investigations. Major aims were (1) to provide for more comprehensive and objective assessments of outcome in children who had suffered this form of early brain disease; (2) to investigate disease and subject factors predictive of outcome; and (3) to enhance awareness of the natural history of this disease throughout the school-age range.

Consideration of previous literature on the effects of Hib meningitis and of other forms of early brain injuries led to the following research hypotheses.

(1) Children who have had Hib meningitis will be affected adversely by the disease. Disease consequences, which will be clearer relative to an appropriate control group than in comparison to normative standards, will include neurological sequelae; deficiencies on tests of cognitive ability; depressed academic skills and poor school performance; and problems in behavioral adjustment, social competence, and adaptive functioning. Cognitive deficits will be apparent on the WISC-R, with greater depression of Performance IQ than of Verbal IQ. Neuropsychological tasks with particular sensitivity to disease effects will be those that have proven most discriminating in previous research (i.e., tests of learning and memory, abstract reasoning, perceptual-motor skill, psychomotor speed, and attention). Other outcome measures will be less consistently affected by disease due to the moderating influence of environmental factors.

Children who have had Hib meningitis will perform below expectations not only as a group, but also in terms of a greater prevalence of learning and behavior handicaps. Indications of these handicaps are scores or ratings that would be considered clinically abnormal on measures of academic skill, school performance, behavior, or social/adaptational competence. Greater than expected rates of grade repetitions or special educational placements provide additional evidence of educational difficulties. Consistent with previous findings, the children will not exhibit a common or single pattern of deficits. Severely affected children, such as those who manifest neurological sequelae, may have multiple deficits. However, sequelae will not be limited to those with abnormal neurological status, and many children will show more isolated impairments that will vary from child to child.

(2) Sequelae will vary in relation to disease characteristics. Although the evidence is by no means clear, it is presumed that neurological insults that occur secondary to Hib meningitis will vary in degree. Brain damage may be severe in some instances but minimal or even nonexistent in other cases. If so, and if more severe insults result in more serious sequelae, then outcomes for a group of children who have had this disease will tend to be skewed, with a greater frequency of adverse outcomes than one would expect in a "normal" sample. In addition, sequelae may be evident for only a portion of the cases and may be more pronounced for some measures of outcome than for others.

Taking disease characteristics as a gauge of the degree of brain insult, and lacking other more direct measures of brain status, sequelae will be more severe and pervasive in association with the following: acute-phase neurological complications (e.g., seizures, coma, hearing loss, cranial nerve abnormalities, motor deficits); more protracted course of illness (i.e., longer interval between onset of symptoms and treatment, longer in-hospital fever duration, longer hospitalization); and more deviant laboratory findings (e.g., higher CSF protein, lower CSF white cell count, lower hemoglobin, and lower CSF/blood glucose ratio). These disease variables will account for variance in outcomes within the group of children who had disease, controlling for either social/environmental factors or the performances of control children.

(3) Sequelae also will vary in relation to subject characteristics. Identification of risks requires conjoint consideration of both disease factors and subject characteristics. Specifically, sequelae of meningitis will be greater the younger the child's age at illness; the older the child at the time of testing; in males compared to females; and the greater the degree of social disadvantage, as suggested by the double hazard hypothesis. The moderating influences of these variables will be evident in terms of their tendencies to compound disease effects. The influence of subject characteristics also will vary within the postmeningitis group. Specifically, children who had a more severe form of the disease will be affected more by subject characteristics than children who had been less severely ill.

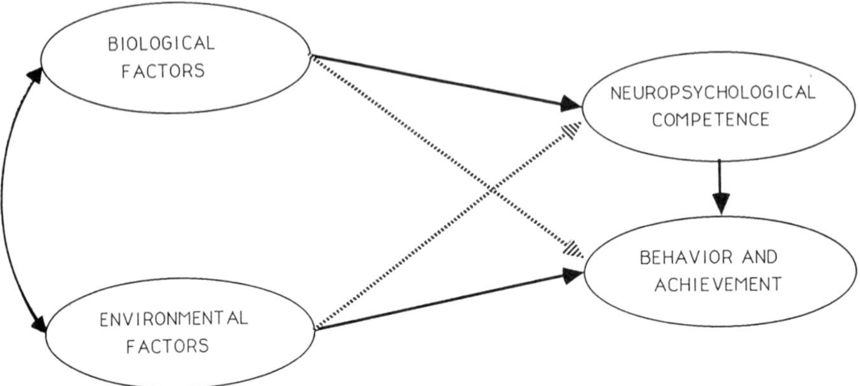

Fig. 3.3. Conceptual model for study of the consequences of early brain disease.

Conceptual Framework

The conceptual framework underlying formulation of these hypotheses is illustrated in Figure 3.3. According to this conceptualization, developmental outcomes following early brain insults are appreciated best in terms of relationships between four constructs: biological factors, environmental factors, neuropsychological competencies, and behavior and achievement.

The construct labeled *biological factors* represents measures of brain insult, as assessed by the presence versus absence of the disease, disease severity, or indices of the type, extent, or location of neuropathology. Other information about the child's medical history (e.g., prenatal and perinatal complications, history of head injury, or other neurological disorder) is also pertinent in assessing this construct.

Environmental factors are assessed in terms of socioeconomic status and family size, as well as more proximal measures of the child's social environment. Measures of the latter sort include parent characteristics (e.g., parental attitudes and psychopathology), parent–child interactions, family social supports and resources, life events, and other aspects of the family environment (Rutter, 1977). Recent research suggests that these variables are of particular relevance in accounting for behavioral outcomes of chronic illness or disability (Breslau, Staruch, & Mortimer, 1982; Crnic, Friedrich, & Greenberg, 1983; Crnic, Greenberg, Ragozin, Robinson, & Basham, 1983). The likelihood that one environmental variable may be moderated by another means that environmental factors will not always have direct effects on outcomes (Crnic, Greenberg, et al., 1983). Nevertheless, prediction will be facilitated by efforts to assess as many of these influences as possible.

Neuropsychological competencies constitute those outcomes that are evaluated by means of performance on tests of cognitive ability. Measures subsumed under this construct satisfy at least one of three criteria: (1) they are sensitive to the presence of brain insults; (2) they help portray the nature of the effects of brain injury on cognitive development; or (3) they are predictive of other, more ecologically meaningful aspects of childhood functioning (Taylor, 1984, 1988; Taylor & Fletcher, in press). Measures that tap information processing skills are distinguished from assessments of accumulated knowledge. The reason for this is that brain disease may have more direct effects on processing skills. Tests that assess acquired knowledge, in contrast, may be more subject to compensatory influences (Rourke, 1982; Taylor, 1984).

The final construct, referred to as *behavior and achievement*, represents outcomes that are ecologically significant, or that directly reflect the child's adaptation at home or school. This area of assessment consists of (1) parent or teacher reports or ratings concerning the child's behavior or academic performance; (2) direct testing of academic skills or classroom observation; and (3) collection of information regarding the child's educational history (e.g., grade repetitions, special educational placements). Outcomes in this category are construed as highly dependent on social and experiential factors.

As shown in Figure 3.3, biological factors are postulated to influence behavior via their effects on neuropsychological competence (see pathway of solid arrows from biological factors to neuropsychological competence to behavior and achievement). The model also allows for effects of biological factors on behavior that are not mediated by neuropsychological deficits, as indicated by hatched arrows (e.g., by direct effects of brain injury on behavior or by disruptions in behavior or social interactions caused by the illness that are perpetuated in spite of neuropsychological recovery) (Rutter, 1977).

The model further presupposes, along with Kopp and Krakow (1983), that appreciation of biological risks requires concomitant consideration of social and developmental influences on the child. Although specific neuropsychological functions are not viewed as immune from social and experiential influences, these environmental factors are assumed to be much more strongly associated with the child's behavior and achievement. Relationships between environmental and biological factors are acknowledged in the curved arrow joining these two constructs. Although not shown in Figure 3.3, the model also recognizes the importance of follow-up of children over time, to determine if the manifestations of disease change with age and to examine associations between past and present functioning.

Pilot Investigation

The foregoing hypotheses and conceptual framework were tested first in a pilot study conducted at the Children's Hospital of Pittsburgh (Taylor et al., 1984). To explore the nature of neurodevelopmental sequelae of Hib meningitis and the predictive validity of both disease and social variables, a group of 24 children who had contracted this disease 6 to 8 years earlier were recruited from consecutive hospital admissions between 1973 and 1975. Criteria for selection were that the postmeningitis, or index, child be in at least the first grade, that he or she have a school-age sibling, and that the child's family live in reasonable proximity of the medical center. All but one of the eligible children participated. Siblings, who were chosen to control for genetic and environmental background factors, were those closest in age to the index children and had no history of neurological problems. Mean age at testing for the index and sibling groups were 8.8 and 11.8, respectively.

Evaluations of the index–sibling pairs were completed in a single half-day session. The children were tested in tandem by psychometricians who were kept blind whenever possible as to the child's group assignment (index or sibling). Testing consisted of the WISC-R; neuropsychological assessment of language abilities, memory, perceptual-motor skill, and attention; and measures of academic achievement. Portions of the test battery were counterbalanced to control for potential fatigue or warm-up effects, and the order of administration of the individual neuropsychological tasks was randomized for each child. Ratings of behavior and temperament, along with information on sociodemographic factors and medical history, were collected from parents while their children were being tested. Data on the acute phase of illness were extracted from medical records.

One of the major findings of this pilot study was that 5 of the 24 index children (21%) manifested neurological sequelae; 1 with mild mental retardation in combination with a chronic seizure disorder; 2 with sensorineural hearing impairment; and 2 with mild hemiparesis. These 5 children performed more poorly on the whole than children who were neurologically normal.

Although mean WISC-R Verbal IQ (VIQ), Performance IQ (PIQ), and Full Scale IQ (FSIQ) fell within the average range for both groups, the index group scored significantly below their siblings on PIQ and FSIQ. Visual inspection of the distribution of FSIQs in the two groups indicated a slight downward shift in the IQs of the index cases relative to sibling IQs. IQs of less than 90 were twice as common in the postmeningitis group than in siblings (i.e., 6 vs. 3 children, respectively). The subgroup of index children with neurological sequelae tended to score below the remainder of the group on IQ, but group differences were significant even for the subset of 19 index cases without sequelae. Consistent with expectations, PIQ was significantly lower than VIQ for the postmeningitis group only.

A tally of the number of deficient performances (i.e., scores at least 2 standard deviations below age norms) observed in tests of specific neuropsychological functions indicated a higher rate of impairment for the index group than for siblings. As in the case of IQ differences, this effect was reliable even when analysis was restricted to the cases without neurological sequelae. Significant differences in favor of the siblings were found on tasks requiring (1) the ability to follow orally presented, multistep directions (Token Test); (2) motor integrity and perceptual-motor skill and speed (Grooved Pegboard Test and an aggregate measure of "soft" neurological status); and (3) memorization of a supraspan list of words (Verbal Selective Reminding Test). The groups did not differ, however, on tests of picture naming, design copying, sentence construction, or phonological analysis. Measures of academic achievement and parent ratings of behavior and temperament also failed to distinguish index children from siblings.

Multiple linear regression analyses revealed that several of the medical variables were predictive of outcome in the postmeningitis group, with R^2 ranging from .19 to .68. Poorer test performances were associated with lower CSF glucose, younger age at admission, longer fever duration, and higher CSF protein. Further confirmation of a relationship between medical risk and outcome was provided by examining the medical records of the children who had suffered outright neurological sequelae. Three of these children had seizures with their illness, four were 7 months of age or younger at the time of illness, and three had symptoms for an extensive period before being hospitalized. There were too few children in this subset to permit statistical analysis, but these risks were not as frequently noted among the remainder of the group.

A final result was the tendency for children with developmental handicaps—identified on the basis of neurological sequelae, subnormal IQ, or academic underachievement—to have siblings who were likewise handicapped. Although 11 of the index cases (46%) were handicapped by these criteria, so were 7 of the siblings (29%). The odds that the index child would have a handicap appeared considerably raised when the sibling was handicapped: in 5 of the 7 pairs in which the sibling was handicapped, the index child was also handicapped. Sell (1983) and Tejani et al. (1982) observed similar concordances between postmeningitis children and their siblings. Such intrafamilial resemblances support the use of sibling controls and underscore the importance of taking social and family influences into account in evaluating disease consequences (Taylor, 1984, 1987).

The findings of the Pittsburgh study confirmed the existence of sequelae, demonstrated that certain measures of outcome were more affected than other measures, and showed that some of the variability in outcomes could be predicted from medical and family background factors. The absence of differences in academic achievement was puzzling, especially in view of a 7-point difference in FSIQ. Remarkably, a follow-up study by Feldman and Michaels (1988) revealed that these children continued to make normal academic progress 3 to 4 years later. In general, the results indicated that disease consequences were more benign than had been thought, at least for the majority of these children. This pilot work also argued against any simplistic assumptions about sparing of functions following early brain insults. Some skills may be more spared than others, and the vulnerability of the child to developmental handicaps is likely a function of multiple biological and psychosocial influences. Disease morbidity is difficult to assess without consideration of non-disease factors.

Current Methods

Procedures and Sampling Strategy

Our present research program was initiated to confirm these findings and to elaborate further on the manner in which meningitis affects development of school-age children. The major goal was to recruit a much larger number of children over a wider age range and to follow these children for 3 years. Testing procedures were much the same as those used in the pilot investigation. Changes in method were the following. First, each child's hearing was screened with a portable audiometer prior to testing to be sure that any hearing impairments had been identified. Second, an updated neuropsychological battery was administered. Third, more data on behavior and achievement were obtained, including both teacher and parent ratings, assessments of adaptive behaviors, and information regarding each child's educational history. Fourth, social and familial factors were evaluated more comprehensively. Fifth, more extensive reviews of medical history and hospital records were undertaken to examine disease course and subsequent health status. Independent and dependent variables are listed in Table 3.1.

Beginning in 1985, children were recruited from three Canadian children's hospitals (Montreal Children's Hospital, The Children's Hospital of Eastern Ontario, and The Hospital for Sick Children in Toronto). Attempts were made to recruit all eligible children who were treated at these three hospitals from 1972 to 1984. Eligibility criteria were (1) history of a single episode of Hib meningitis; (2) age between 6 and 14 years at the time of the initial testing; (3) no evidence of other neurological disease either prior to or following the meningitis; and (4) residence within the greater metropolitan areas surrounding these hospitals. To enhance the applicability of test norms, particularly as the project was carried out in bilingual cities, an additional restriction was that the children's education had to have been primarily in English for at least 1 year.

Most of the 392 eligible children who did not participate could not be traced from information in the charts. The remainder of those who did not take part were attending non-English schools, had histories of other neurological disorders, or declined to participate due to busy schedules,

Table 3.1. Variables in the present study.

Independent variables

I. Demographic
- Age at testing
- Gender

II. Social
- Hollingshead Two Factor Index of Socioeconomic Status (SES)
- Home Environment Questionnaire (HEQ)
  - Achievement
  - Aggression—home
  - Aggression—external
  - Aggression—total
  - Supervision
  - Change
  - Affiliation
  - Separation
  - Sociability
  - Socioeconomic Status (SES)
- Life Events Questionnaire
  - Positive events
  - Negative events

III. Medical
- Age at admission
- Presence or absence of a neurological complication
- Length of hospital stay
- Duration of fever
- Time between onset of symptoms and hospitalization
- CSF/blood glucose ratio
- CSF white cell
- CSF protein
- Hemoglobin

Dependent variables

I. Intelligence
- WISC-R
  - Performance IQ
  - Verbal IQ
  - Full Scale IQ

II. Academic Achievement
- WRAT-R
  - Reading
  - Spelling
  - Arithmetic
- Gilmore Oral Reading Test
  - Accuracy
  - Comprehension

III. Neuropsychological Skills
- Language Abilities
  - Token Test
  - Word Fluency
- Psychomotor Skills
  - Grooved Pegboard Test
  - Beery-Buktenika Test of Visual-Motor Integration

continued

Table 3.1. *Continued*

Dependent variables
Memory
Verbal Selective Reminding Test
Nonverbal Selective Reminding Test
Attention
Underlining Test
Continuous Performance Test
Contingency Naming Test
Abstract Reasoning
Cattell Culture Fair Test, Scale 2
IV. Behavioral Adjustment: Child Behavior Checklist and Teacher's Report Form
V. School Performance
School Performance Scale, Teacher's Report Form
Number of hours per week of special educational assistance, year of testing
Parent's Rating of Educational Progress[a]
VI. Adaptive Behavior
Vineland Adaptive Behavior Scales

Key: WISC-R, Wechsler Intelligence Scale for Children–Revised; WRAT-R, Wide Range Achievement Test–Revised.

[a] Ratings obtained by having parents estimate school progress for all years attended (0 = poor, 1 = fair, 2 = good) and averaging across years.

disinterest, or transportation difficulties. A total of 127 children participated (25 from Montreal, 43 from Ottawa, and 59 from Toronto). In 97 of these cases, a nearest age sibling was also invited to take part. All of these siblings were biologically related to the index child, had negative neurological histories, and had been educated primarily in English for at least 1 year.

The proportion of males and females was approximately equal in each group. The average age in years of the index and sibling groups at the time of the initial testing was 9.7 (SD = 2.3) and 11.6 (SD = 2.7), respectively. Mean SES for the 127 families on the Hollingshead Two-Factor Index was 61.9 (SD = 27.1). Mean occupational status and parent education both fell at midscale (3.3, SD = 1.6 for occupation; 3.0, SD = 1.5 for education). Mean sibship size was 2.7 (SD = 1.1). Neither sample characteristics nor measures of acute-phase disease severity differed by test site. Time postillness, which averaged 8.2 years (SD = 2.5), was highly related to age at testing ($r = .88$, $p < .001$). Neither variable, however, was correlated with age at illness. Comparison of the index children to candidates for the study whose families declined to take part failed to reveal any differences in disease severity. Disease severity also failed to distinguish the subgroups of index cases with and without sibling matches.

Initial evaluations were the same for the children in both groups. The index cases, but not siblings, were then reevaluated annually for two consecutive years. Procedures identical to those used in the initial testing were readministered to these children, their parents, and teachers at each assessment. Data collection was completed recently and analysis is ongoing.

Design and Analysis

Plans for analysis were guided by the three essential components of the design: (1) comparison of index cases to sibling controls on a multitude of outcome measures; (2) search for variables predictive of variability in outcomes within the index group; and (3) longitudinal follow-up of the index children to investigate stability and change over time. Each of these elements is discussed in turn for the purposes of reviewing our analytic methods and of highlighting methodological issues encountered in conducting this type of research.

Comparison of Index Cases to Siblings

Two methods of comparison were used to determine if there were differences in outcome between index cases and siblings (Hypothesis 1). The first method involved comparison of the total sample of 127 index cases to the 97 siblings, adjusting for any group differences in social factors or sex distribution via covariance analyses. To minimize Type I error in a fashion that would not be overly restrictive with respect to our ability to recognize meaningful differences, we divided outcome measures on a priori grounds into the domains listed in Table 3.1. The justification for partitioning outcomes is that each domain represents a different developmental construct, for which a separate hypothesis could be posed regarding disease effects. Differences in the domains of intelligence and adaptive behavior were examined by means of group t tests on FSIQ and the Vineland Adaptive Behavior Composite, respectively. Multivariate analyses of variance (MANOVAs) were employed to investigate group differences in the other domains. MANOVAs allowed us to take the several parameters comprising these domains into account simultaneously while maintaining acceptable subject to variable ratios (Timm, 1977). Groups were also compared in terms of individual parameters within domains (e.g., VIQ and PIQ within the domain of intelligence and parent and teacher ratings in the domain of behavioral adjustment), with Bonferroni adjustments made in alpha level (.05) as suggested by Bray and Maxwell (1982) and by Huberty and Morris (1989). To discover if sequelae could be identified even in children who were not at risk due to hearing loss or other overt physical disorder, analyses were conducted both with and without data from index cases who had concurrent neurological sequelae.

The second approach was to restrict analyses to the 97 index cases with sibling controls and to employ multivariate Hotelling's T^2 tests (Tatsuoka, 1971) on the index–sibling difference scores. In support of the latter

Table 3.2. Index–sibling test score correlations.

Domain and test	r	Domain and test	r
I. Intelligence		Social Competence	.53***
WISC-R		Teacher's Report Form	
Verbal IQ	.47***	Behavior Problems	.18*
Performance IQ	.52***	School Adjustment	.37**
Full Scale IQ	.53***	V. School Performance	
II. Academic Achievement		Teacher's Report Form–School Performance	.38**
WRAT-R		Parent's Rating of Educational Progress	.25**
Reading	.47***	Number of hours per week of special educational assistance, year of testing	.02
Spelling	.17	VI. Adaptive Behavior	
Arithmetic	.15	Vineland Adaptive Behavior Scales	
Gilmore Oral Reading Test		Socialization	.46***
Accuracy	.35**	Communication	.35***
Comprehension	.28**	Daily Living	.41***
III. Neuropsychological Skills[a]		Adaptive Behavior Composite	.50***
Language Abilities	.24*		
Psychomotor Skills	.28**		
Memory	.28**		
Attention	.26**		
Abstract Reasoning	.27**		
IV. Behavioral Adjustment			
Child Behavior Checklist			
Behavior Problems	.55***		

[a] Composite scores used in calculating correlations for neuropsychological domain defined as average z scores of test parameters comprising each subdomain.
* $p < .05$.
** $p < .01$.
*** $p < .001$.

approach, there were robust correlations between pair members across all outcome domains (see Table 3.2). Paired comparisons proved to be a powerful means for investigating disease consequences. The choice of siblings as controls was therefore well advised.

Both methods of comparison utilized outcome measures that had been age-standardized prior to analyses. The only exceptions were number of hours of special educational assistance and parent ratings of educational progress (see Table 3.1). Because norms that spanned the age range of our sample were not available for most of the neuropsychological tests, sibling data were used for this purpose. Following a procedure employed in previous neuropsychological research, regression methods were first applied to find the linear combination of age and sex polynomials that best predicted each dependent variable. Performance was then standardized in terms of the difference, in standard deviation units between observed and predicted raw score values (Decker & DeFries, 1981; Ryan, Morrow, Bromet, & Parkinson, 1987).

The two groups were additionally compared in terms of the frequencies of cases for which test findings or parent judgments suggested at least mild problems in cognitive development, learning, behavior, or adaptive functioning. Comparisons of this nature shed light on the clinical significance of disease consequences. The latter "handicapping conditions" were defined as (1) low WISC-R FSIQ (<80); (2) impaired performance on one or more of the other neuropsychological tests (score at least 2 standard deviations below sibling-based predictions); (3) low WRAT-R standard score (<80); (4) grade repetition; (5) past or current placement in special educational program for a learning problem; (6) Internalizing or Externalizing *T* score in the clinical range (>63) on either the Child Behavior Checklist or Teacher's Report Form; and (7) low Vineland Adaptive Behavior Composite (<80). Corresponding to the two methods described, both chi-square analyses (using data for all subjects) and McNemar tests (using index–sibling pairs) were conducted to determine if handicapping conditions were more prevalent for index children than for siblings. Other reasons for identifying individual handicaps were to test the notion that sequelae would vary across children, to investigate comorbidity, and to determine whether children with handicaps were different from those without handicaps in disease severity or subject characteristics.

Predictors of Outcome

Regression techniques were used to identify predictors of individual post-meningitis outcomes. Hierarchical multiple linear regression models were employed when the outcome measure was a continuous variable and logistic regression models were used for categorical outcomes (e.g., repeated a grade, special educational placement) (Bock, 1975; Cohen & Cohen, 1983). One objective of these analyses was to discover whether indices of disease severity accounted for variability in outcomes that could not be explained by factors unrelated to the illness (Hypothesis 2). The other objective was to determine whether subject characteristics moderated disease effects (Hypothesis 3). Procedures for minimizing Type I error were similar to those used in analyzing index–sibling differences.

Two methods of analysis were employed. The first, or unmatched, method for testing Hypothesis 2 included data from all 127 index cases. The initial step in this approach was to conduct a series of stepwise multiple regressions to identify the social/familial predictors of post-meningitis outcomes. Outcomes were represented in these analyses either by single scores or, in the case of neuropsychological domains other than IQ, by domain composites. The latter composites were defined by averaging *z* scores across the individual measures comprising each domain. The results of these analyses, presented in Table 3.3, indicate which variables were the best predictors. Results also demonstrate that a substantial proportion of the variability in outcome measures was predicted by background social and family circumstances (see R^2 values in

Table 3.3. Social variables predictive of outcomes in 127 index children.

Domain and measure	Social set	R^2
I. Intelligence		
WISC-R		
Verbal IQ	Hollingshead SES; HEQ-SES	.31***
Performance IQ	HEQ-SES, Change, Aggression Home, Achievement	.21***
Full Scale IQ	HEQ-SES, Change	.25***
II. Academic Achievement		
WRAT-R		
Reading	Hollingshead SES	.21***
Spelling	Hollingshead SES; Negative Life Events	.19***
Arithmetic	Hollingshead SES; HEQ-Supervision	.14**
Gilmore Oral Reading Test		
Accuracy	HEQ-Sociability, Achievement; Negative and Positive Life Events	.33***
Comprehension	Negative Life Events; HEQ-Achievement	.24***
III. Neuropsychological Skills[a]		
Language Abilities	Hollingshead SES; Positive Life Events; HEQ-Supervision	.15**
Psychomotor Skills		NS
Memory	Hollingshead SES; HEQ-SES	.09*
Attention		NS
Abstract Reasoning	Hollingshead SES	.10**
IV. Behavioral Adjustment		
CBCL		
Internalizing	HEQ-Aggression Total, Aggression Home; Negative Life Events	.42***
Externalizing	HEQ-Aggression Total, Aggression Home; Hollingshead SES	.38***
Total Behavior Problems	HEQ-Aggression Total, Aggression Home	.40***
Social Competence	Positive Life Events; HEQ-SES	.35***
TRF		
Internalizing	Positive Life Events; HEQ-Change	.11**
Externalizing	HEQ-Aggression Total	.10*
Total Behavior Problems	HEQ-Aggression Total	.09*
School Adjustment	Positive Life Events	.13**
V. School Performance		
TRF		
School Performance	Positive and Negative Life Events	.23***
Parent's Rating of Educational Progress	HEQ-Achievement	.14**
VI. Adaptive Behavior		
Vineland Adaptive Behavior Scales		
Communication	HEQ-SES; Positive Life Events; Gender	.38***
Socialization	HEQ-Sociability; Gender; Age at testing; Hollingshead SES	.31***
Daily Living	HEQ-Aggression Total; Negative Life Events; Gender	.22***
Adaptive Behavior Composite	HEQ-SES; Positive Life Events; Gender	.36***

Key: WISC-R, Wechsler Intelligence Scale for Children-Revised; WRAT-R, Wide Range Achievement Test-Revised; CBCL, Child Behavior Checklist; TRF, Teacher's Report Form; HEQ, Home Environment Questionnaire; NS, Nonsignificant.

[a] Composite scores used in calculating correlations for neuropsychological domain defined as average *z* scores of test parameters comprising each subdomain.

this table). The social/familial variables that accounted for significant variability in each outcome were then forced to enter the hierarchical regression equation as covariates, followed by entry of all measures of disease severity by set. In cases where disease severity accounted for significant additional variance in an outcome, each of the individual measures of disease severity was entered singly, after the covariates, in search of important individual predictors.

The unmatched method for testing Hypothesis 3 entailed prediction of outcomes for the total groups of both index cases and siblings. In this instance, each of the outcomes was regressed first on main effect terms. Factors included in these analyses were presence/absence of disease, age at testing, sex, and social/familial status. For the purposes of these analyses, social/familial status was represented by a single index (e.g., SES or a z score composite of the best set of social predictors). Terms representing the interaction of group with each of the subject characteristics were then tested.

Matched-sample methods for testing Hypotheses 2 and 3 were similar to those just described. The major difference was that scores for index cases were included in the analysis only when siblings' scores were also available, and the siblings' scores were entered as covariates prior to the inclusion of any of the independent variables. In this manner, the effects of disease severity and the moderating influences of subject characteristics could be examined in relation to "sibling-adjusted" outcome. The virtue of this second method was that it allowed for tighter control of background variables, especially genetic factors.

An alternative, within-group (index cases only) approach for exploring interactions of disease effects with subject characteristics was to employ disease severity, rather than group membership, as the disease variable. Following this approach, outcomes for the 127 index cases were first examined as a function of main effects for disease severity and subject characteristics. Terms representing interactions of each of the measures of disease severity with each of the four subject factors were then entered into the regression model.

Longitudinal Follow-Up

Although our examination of the longitudinal data collected in Years 2 and 3 of the project is not yet complete, repeated measures MANOVAs will serve as our primary analytic tool (Bock, 1975; Timm, 1977). Following the suggestions of O'Brien and Kaiser (1985), changes over time will be examined in terms of difference scores between outcomes in Year 2 compared to Year 1 and in Year 3 compared to Year 1. These two difference scores will then be tested against the constant to determine whether there are significant changes across the 3 years. Our hypothesis is that performances will decline relative to age standards, at least in some outcome domains (e.g., academic achievement). Differential change as a function of disease severity and subject characteristics will be investigated by incorporating these variables into the model. We also will examine change in relation to other variables—notably, the presence/absence of neurological sequelae and indications of initial handicaps. Hierarchical linear modeling (Bryk & Raudenbush, 1987) constitutes another promising method for study of longitudinal change, in which raw scores are used to estimate within-subject growth trajectories. Between-subject variables that account for differences in these trajectories are then identified.

The relative stability in childhood functioning is also of interest. Intraclass correlations will be used to assess reliability of performance across test occasions. Disease or subject factors associated with declining functioning will be studied by means of log linear methods (Green, 1988) or, alternatively, by searching for factors that discriminate children making little or no progress from children whose progress is more age-appropriate.

The major advantage of this component of the design is the opportunity it affords for more powerful study of differences in outcome as a function of age at testing (Baltes, 1968). Rogosa, Brandt, and Zimowski (1982) make an especially strong appeal for analysis of longitudinal change. They also stress the importance of obtaining more than two observations per subject. The longitudinal analyses to be performed will provide important new information on the natural history of development postmeningitis and on the importance of analyses of change in child neuropsychology (Fletcher et al., 1990; Francis, Fletcher, Maxwell, & Satz, 1989).

Two potential weaknesses of this element of the design relate to sample attrition and practice effects that accrue with repeated annual administrations of psychometric testing. Although attrition was insubstantial (only 7% between Years 1 and 2 and 1% between Years 2 and 3), it will be necessary to compare systematically those children who left the study early to the remainder of the group to check for any differences in sample composition across testings. Because practice effects will tend to obscure evidence for progressively greater sequelae with age, it is equally important to consider these effects in interpreting longitudinal changes. Following a procedure used by Hakuta (1987), practice effects will be estimated by comparing the performances of subsets of similarly aged children distinguished in terms of their previous testing experience.

Preliminary Findings

Hypothesis 1: Overall Disease Consequences

The incidence of neurological sequelae in the total postmeningitis sample was comparable to that observed in several other investigations (Feigin et al., 1976; Jadavji et al., 1986; Lebel et al., 1988; Sell, 1983; Taylor et al.,

1984). Eighteen (14%) of these children had neurological sequelae that failed to resolve within 6 weeks after their discharge from the hospital. Sixteen children from this subgroup (13% of the total sample) continued to evidence sequelae concurrent with our testing. Neurological sequelae took the form of neurosensory hearing impairment and other cranial nerve abnormalities, seizures, hemiparesis, and ataxia (Mills, MacDonald, Gold, & Taylor, 1988; Taylor, Lean, Michaels, & Mills, 1987; Taylor, Mills, Watters, & Kormos, 1988).

In view of the neurological consequences of the disease, there were surprisingly few indications of disease effects in other areas. Although the index group scored more poorly than the siblings on virtually all measures, differences were small. The only domains in which index children performed significantly less well than siblings on group comparison were intelligence (WISC-R Performance and Full Scale IQs), memory, academic achievement (WRAT-R Reading and Spelling, and Gilmore Accuracy and Comprehension), and adaptive behavior (Vineland Communication Scale). Results of the paired comparisons were much the same (Taylor et al., 1990). Site of testing was unrelated to these differences. As anticipated, most of these differences remained significant even when index children with concurrent neurologic sequelae were excluded from analysis.

Although the relative incidence of handicapping conditions was also greater in the index children compared to siblings, the only significant difference was in the frequency of current special educational placements (see Table 3.4). Again, findings were similar when comparisons were restricted to index–sibling pairs (Taylor et al., 1990).

No one handicap or pattern of handicaps was characteristic of the children in either group. There was a general tendency for concurrence of low IQs, academic underachievement, and problematic educational histories (e.g., special educational placements, grade repetitions), but isolated deficits also were apparent. Most children with academic handicaps or behavior problems had normal IQs.

As seen in Table 3.5, many children from both groups also manifested specific neuropsychological impairments. These impairments ranged widely and were usually associated with normal IQ. Due partly to the greater number of tests in this area, attention deficits were more common than other neuropsychological dysfunctions. Nevertheless, index children were significantly more likely than siblings to have one or more impaired scores on the attention tasks (37% vs. 13%, $p < .001$). The relative frequency of multiple areas of neuropsychological impairment was also higher in the index group (13% vs. 4%, $p < .05$).

Hypothesis 2: Relationship of Disease Severity to Outcome

The distributions of WISC-R Full Scale IQs for the sibling-matched index cases and siblings are presented in Figure 3.4. Inspection of this figure

Table 3.4. Incidence of findings suggestive of a handicapping condition in 127 index children vs. 97 siblings.

Condition	Criteria	Index	Sibling	χ^2
Low IQ	WISC-R full scale IQ < 80	6 (5%)	0 (0%)	3.07
Limited academic skills	At least one WRAT-R standard score < 80	29 (23%)	17 (18%)	.38
Poor school achievement	Grade repetition	19 (15%)	12 (13%)	.14
Need for special educational assistance	Past special educational assistance	35 (28%)	20 (21%)	1.20
	Current special educational assistance	35 (28%)	12 (13%)	6.64[a]
Behavior problems	Internalizing or externalizing—score in the clinical range on the CBCL or TRF	24 (19%)	10 (13%)	.49
Poor adaptive functioning	Vineland Adaptive Behavior Composite < 80	10 (8%)	9 (9%)	.02

Key: WISC-R, Wechsler Intelligence Scale for Children–Revised; WRAT-R, Wide Range Achievement Test–Revised; CBCL, Child Behavior Checklist; TRF, Teacher's Report Form.

[a] Significant.

Table 3.5. Rates of neuropsychological impairments in 127 index children and 97 siblings

Deficit area (s)	Index group[a]	Sibling group[a]
(1) Language Ability	1 (1)	3 (3)
(2) Psychomotor Skills	3 (2)	3 (3)
(3) Memory	2 (1)	6 (6)
(4) Attention[b]	31 (24)	11 (11)
(5) Abstract Reasoning	0 (0)	0 (0)
(1) and (2)	1 (1)	0 (0)
(1) and (3)	1 (1)	1 (1)
(1) and (4)	5 (4)	0 (0)
(1) and (5)	0 (0)	1 (1)
(2) and (3)	2 (1)	0 (0)
(2) and (4)	4 (3)	0 (0)
(3) and (4)	2 (1)	0 (0)
(4) and (5)	1 (1)	2 (2)
(1), (2), and (4)	1 (1)	0 (0)
(2), (3), and (4)	2 (1)	0 (0)
(1), (2), (4), and (5)	1 (1)	0 (0)
Total with deficits[b]	57 (45)	27 (28)

[a] Number of children as percentage of total given is in parenthesis.

[b] Differences with respect to attention and Total significant ($p < .05$).

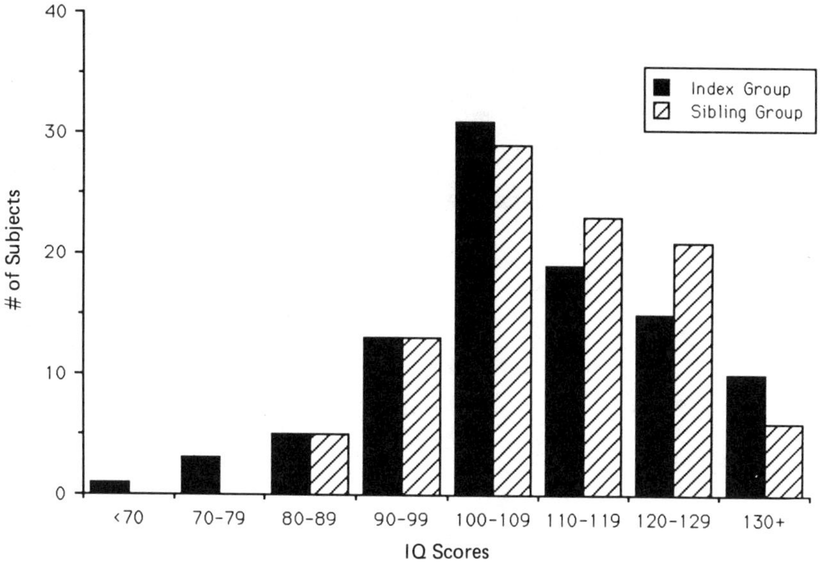

Fig. 3.4. Distribution of Full Scale IQ scores (WISC-R).

suggests that the anticipated skewness in the distribution of index IQs is present in this sample. A downward shift is also evident within the higher ranges of IQ.

With background factors controlled by covarying for either social/familial variables (total sample) or sibling score (matched sample), more adverse outcomes were associated with acute-phase neurological complications, in-hospital fever duration, CSF white cell count, and CSF/blood glucose ratio. As illustrated in Figure 3.5, the presence of a neurological complication had special significance (Taylor et al., 1990). Index–sibling paired differences on the WISC-R, WRAT–R, and Vineland were more marked when analysis was restricted to the 41 pairs in which the index case had a complication (Figure 3.5b) than they were in the overall analysis, differences were virtually nonexistent in the remaining 56 pairs (Figure 3.5a). In 11 of the 41 pairs in which index children had complications, the sibling's IQ exceeded that of the index child by at least 15 points. By comparison, there was only one pair in which the index child's IQ exceeded that of the sibling by this amount ($p < .01$). The discrepancy between WISC-R Verbal and Performance IQ also was marginally significant for this subgroup (respective means of 105 and 101, $p = .08$) but negligible for the remainder of the index children and for siblings.

Exploratory analyses of index children with neurological complications suggested that the type of neurological complication sustained during the acute-phase illness (e.g., whether the child was in coma, had seizures,

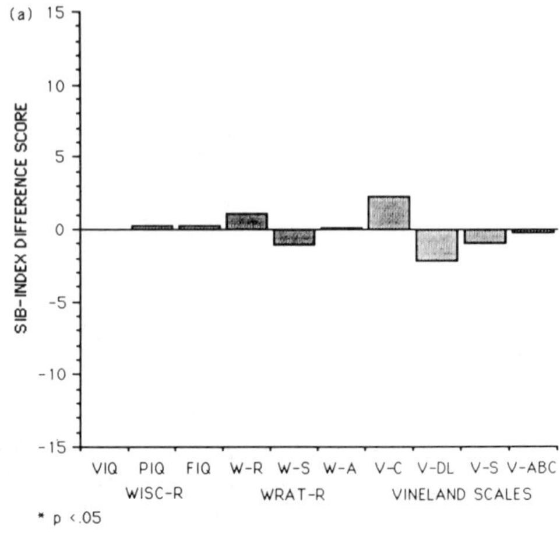

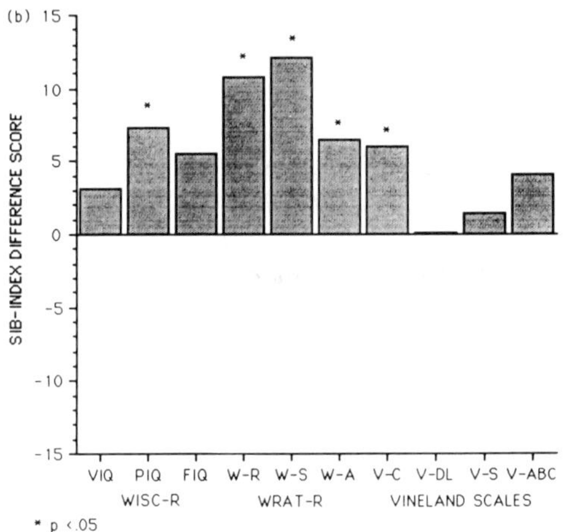

Fig. 3.5. Sibling–index difference scores on tests of intelligence, academic achievement, and adaptive behavior (a) for 56 children without neurological complications and their siblings and (b) for 41 children with neurological complications and their siblings.

Key: WISC-R, Wechsler Intelligence Scale for Children–Revised; VIQ, Verbal IQ; PIQ, Performance IQ; FIQ, Full Scale IQ; WRAT-R, Wide Range Achievement Test–Revised; W-R, WRAT-R Reading; W-S, WRAT-R Spelling; W-A, WRAT-R Arithmetic; V-C, Vineland Communication Domain; V-DL, Vineland Daily Living Domain; V-S, Vineland Socialization Domain; V-ABC, Vineland Adaptive Behavior Composite.

was hemiplegic, or sustained a hearing loss) may be of additional value in predicting eventual outcomes (Taylor et al., 1988). Comparisons of index children with and without handicaps offered converging support for the relevance of neurological complications to outcomes. These comparisons also revealed associations between handicapping conditions and social/familial status.

Hypothesis 3: Subject Characteristics as Moderators of Disease Consequences

Regression analyses involving unmatched groups provided little support for interactions between disease presence/absence and subject characteristics. The only exception was an interaction of group and sex in the prediction of parent ratings of behavior problems. According to further analyses, the basis for this interaction was the fact that female siblings were rated higher in behavior problems than male siblings. For the index children, in contrast, there was a nonsignificant trend in the opposite direction. If sex differences among siblings are viewed as "normative" for this sample, findings offer tentative support for the position that the disease had greater behavioral consequences for males than for females. Of some additional interest was the fact that the inclusion of main effect terms for all subject factors yielded more powerful tests of disease effects. Significant group effects were found not only for IQ, academic achievement, and Vineland Communication, but also for the Vineland Adaptive Behavior Composite and behavior problems.

Clearer evidence in support of the moderating influence of subject characteristics was obtained in regression analyses restricted to the index–sibling pairs. As described earlier, sibling scores served as covariates in these analyses, followed by terms representing main effects for subject characteristics. Significant main effects indicate that outcomes for index children were dependent on subject factors over and above whatever influence these factors had on siblings' scores. Controlling for sibling scores, outcomes for index cases varied with sex, age at testing, and SES (Taylor et al., 1990). Tests for simple effects revealed that both teacher ratings of school adjustment and the Vineland Adaptive Behavior Composite discriminated the index children from their siblings, but only when the index child was male. Older index children showed more prominent behavior problems compared to siblings than did younger index children. Finally, lower SES was predictive of lower WISC-R Verbal IQ for the index cases, lower WRAT-R Spelling and Arithmetic, and lower Vineland Communication and Adaptive Behavior Composite scores. A likely explanation for the moderating effect of SES is that some of the influence of this variable on the index child is not reflected in the sibling's score. The effects of SES do not, in other words, constitute evidence for true interactions of disease effects with environmental factors.

Analyses of variability in outcomes within the index group failed to reveal any interactions between disease severity and subject characteristics. Again, inclusion of main effects for all subject factors improved the precision of the analysis of disease effects. In this case, main effects for disease severity were found for WISC-R Performance and Full Scale IQ; neuropsychological tests of psychomotor skill, memory, attention, and abstract reasoning; WRAT-R Reading and Spelling; and the teacher's rating of school performance.

Conclusions

Preliminary results from the present multicenter study of Hib meningitis expand considerably on pilot findings. The primary thrust of this larger project has been to demonstrate the complexity of evaluating disease outcomes. It is clear that the disease can have adverse effects on development. What is most informative, however, is evidence that disease consequences vary as a function of both the disease process and subject characteristics. An accurate portrayal of sequelae would not have been possible, or at least would have been misleading, had our selection of measures been less broad based, and had both disease and subject factors not been taken into account.

Support for Hypothesis 1 was substantial. Hib meningitis has small but definite adverse consequences across multiple developmental domains. Either all or some subset of the index children had lower reading and spelling skills, were more frequently placed in special educational programs, and were rated by parents and teachers as more deviant in behavior, adjustment, and adaptive functioning. Differences were additionally apparent on a neuropsychological battery. The index group has lower WISC-R Performance and Full Scale IQs, with PIQ marginally lower than VIQ for the subgroup with neurological complications; they scored less well relative to age norms on tests of attention and memory; and they were more likely to exhibit multiple neuropsychological impairments. These findings were evidenced in both paired and unpaired comparisons of the index children and siblings, but they were most clearly documented in analyses that took disease and subject factors into account. Results parallel those of other studies of the effects of childhood brain injuries and suggest that CNS insults have greater or more consistent effects on some cognitive abilities than on others (Levin et al., 1987; Taylor, 1987).

The fact that outcomes for index children and siblings were intercorrelated suggests that siblings served as effective controls for background social and genetic factors. Differences in outcome were therefore most probably CNS-related. Although index children were younger on average than their siblings, sibling rank differed by only one. Furthermore, differences were not confined to pairs in which the sibling was older, as would be expected if birth order effects were responsible for the poorer outcomes of the index group (Belmont & Marolla, 1973). Processes unrelated to the index child's brain status conceivably contributed to the differences observed in this study. Possibilities include adverse effects of hospitalization on the child, differential parental treatment due to perceived vulnerability, or disruptions in parent–child interactions originating from temporary disease effects (Masten & Garmezy, 1985; Peloquin & Davidson, 1989; Rutter, 1985). These alternative explanations appear less plausible, however, when one considers the fact that cognitive abilities were more widely affected than behavior and that aspects of the acute-phase illness were predictive of outcomes in the index group.

Means for the index group were well within the average range in every outcome domain and overall group differences were slight. The index children without acute-phase neurological complications did not manifest later neurological disorders, nor did they differ from siblings in any other respect. Mean index–sibling differences were small even within the subgroup of cases with complications. Siblings outperformed index children in Full Scale IQ (by at least 15 points) in only about one-quarter of the latter pairings. The major implication of these findings is that although group differences belie the severity of sequelae for some individuals, consequences are not nearly as pervasive or devastating as was once believed. The impression that as many as half of the survivors experience long-term consequences (Sell, 1983), which was not substantiated in this investigation, may reflect sampling differences. Based on the present findings, sequelae would be expected to vary with both disease severity and subject characteristics. Other reasons for the lesser morbidity observed in this study may relate to the tighter control that was achieved over nondisease influences on outcome and the more systematic manner in which participants were recruited.

Hypothesis 2 also was confirmed. Disease consequences were clearly dependent on indices of disease severity. Risks for sequelae varied in accordance with the presence/absence of neurological complications, in-hospital fever duration, CSF white cell count, and CSF/blood glucose ratio. Results point to the need to view brain disease in gradations, rather than as all-or-none phenomena, and to be cautious in drawing conclusions based on group findings (Taylor, 1984, 1987). The absence of measurable sequelae in index children without neurological complications is also reminiscent of Rutter's (1982) concept of a "threshold" level of brain insult below which there is no demonstrable behavioral effect. Although one cannot rule out sequelae in all such cases, residual damage typically may be so slight as to have no observable impact. Other possibilities are that these children sustained no permanent neuropathology or were able to compensate fully for their injuries through behavioral substitution or vicarious neural functioning. Detailed neuropathological studies of children who have had Hib meningitis, by means of magnetic resonance imaging or other advanced scanning procedures, would be useful in investigating these alternative possibilities. Direct measurement of neuropathology also might help to target the types of neurological complications that are most predictive of outcome. In-depth neuropathological studies, however, are not routinely performed, and we are aware of no systematic research in this area.

Search for disease factors that would allow more precise determination of risks is ongoing. As might be anticipated on the basis of previous findings, exploratory analyses of the present data suggest that risks for sequelae are dependent on the specific pattern of neurological complications. For example, children who were in coma during their illness or who had persistent seizures appear to be at higher risk for some sequelae than those with hearing impairment or transitory seizures (Klein et al., 1986; Taylor et al., 1988). Preliminary analyses also indicate that sequelae were not confined to those cases manifesting persistent neurological deficits. Group differences were significant even when analysis was restricted to index children with neurological symptoms of less than 6 weeks duration. The latter finding supports previous observations of sequelae in children without concurrent neurological disorder (Taylor et al., 1984) but additionally points to the difficulty one faces in gauging CNS insult from overt symptomatology.

In support of Hypothesis 3, sequelae were related additionally to the index child's age and gender. As anticipated, older index children were rated as having more pronounced behavior problems relative to their siblings than was the case for younger index children (Taylor et al., 1990). The absence of age differences in other outcome domains failed to confirm expectations for age-related decreases in cognitive and academic abilities (Dennis et al., 1987; Nussbaum, Grant, Roman, Poole, & Bigler, 1990; Wills et al., 1990) but corroborated the results of a recent follow-up study of the original Pittsburgh pilot sample (Feldman & Michaels, 1988). The fact that cognitive and academic sequelae did not vary as a function of age suggests that the greater behavior problems of older index children were not due to absolute performance limitations. This pattern of results is more compatible with age differences in what is demanded or tolerated from the child or in motivational status (Kopp, 1983). Another possibility is that some unknown selection bias was responsible for these age effects, as is always the case in cross-sectional research. The age of the index child was not confounded with measures of social status or illness severity. However, more time had passed since discharge for older children, and this may have influenced outcomes in some way. Longitudinal follow-up of the index children will permit a more definitive test of the hypothesis that sequelae will tend to worsen over time, at least for some subset of the index cases.

The observation of greater behavioral effects on males relative to females is consistent with the findings of Breslau et al. (1988) and Parkinson et al. (1981) and can be interpreted in much the same fashion as the age differences. Like the age variable, gender was unrelated to cognitive or academic outcomes, disease severity, or social/familial status. Apparently, males tend to cope with or respond to the cognitive and academic sequelae of the disease in a different manner than females or in ways that are more likely to be perceived as problematic (Breslau et al., 1988; Earls, 1987). Differential neuropathology must also be considered, but it is difficult to reconcile with the specificity of the sex effects and with the absence of sex differences in disease severity.

Results failed to indicate that age at illness or social/familial status was related to disease consequences. The lack of an association between sequelae and age at illness may reflect the sample's relatively advanced mean age at illness (18 months). Alternatively, brain insults may have been so minor in this sample as to preclude meaningful study of the influence of age at injury. Absence of support for the double hazard model, in which the effect of brain damage is hypothesized to be augmented by social disadvantage, can be explained on similar grounds. Although the present results are generally consistent with other findings (Breslau, 1990; Rutter, 1977), the present sample may have had too few children with serious CNS insults to investigate this issue properly. Another possibility is that moderating influences of the environment take place by virtue of transactional interactions between parents and children (Masten & Garmezy, 1985; St. James-Roberts, 1979), a process that would not be measured easily by collecting data retrospectively and by measuring separate characteristics of children and families. Prospective follow-ups of parent–child interactions, such as that undertaken with preterm infants by Greenberg and Crnic (1988), would be required to examine interactions of this sort. Following this research strategy, the child's ultimate development would be considered in relation to both direct effects on the child and indirect effects reflective of family adaptation to the child and the child's impact on the family environment (Crnic, Friedrich, & Greenberg, 1983; Plomin, 1989; Rutter, 1985).

It must be emphasized, however, that social variables were reliable correlates of many aspects of the children's development. In agreement with other research on this topic, social variables were robust predictors of behavior and achievement, and they accounted for significant variance in outcomes independent of disease variables (O'Dougherty, Wright, Garmezy, Loewenson, & Torres, 1983). The fact that measures of life events and family environment accounted for variance in many outcomes not explained by SES argues for broad-based assessments of social/environmental status (Costello, 1989a; Crnic, Greenberg, et al., 1983). The present research program also underscores the importance of social assessments to the determination of disease effects (Birch, 1964; Costello,

1989; Hebb, 1949; Rutter, 1977, 1982; Smith, Delves, Lansdown, Clayton, & Graham, 1983; Taylor, 1984; Wolff, 1981). Had care not been taken to measure social variables, or to control for background social and genetic factors, it would have been impossible to isolate the effects of the disease itself. The sizable number of siblings with handicapping conditions or neuropsychological impairments indicates that developmental deficiencies are not uncommon in children without frank brain disease (see Tables 3.4 and 3.5) and that failure to consider baseline expectations would tend to inflate estimates of disease effects.

One of the most theoretically significant findings of this investigation is the evidence it provides for the separate influences of nature and nurture on psychological development. Consistent with the conceptual framework depicted in Figure 3.3, brain disease was predictive of neuropsychological competencies, which in turn were related to ecologically meaningful aspects of behavior and achievement (Taylor & Schatschneider, 1990). Outcomes most uniformly related to brain disease were Performance IQ and other neuropsychological tests that tap active information processing abilities. Social factors, in contrast, were better predictors of Verbal IQ, achievement, and behavioral adjustment. Results generally support a distinction between biologically based functions, considered to be relatively insensitive to external influences, and functions that are subject to substantial "shaping" by the individual's environment and learning history (Taylor & Fletcher, 1990).

A variety of other research findings offer further support for such a distinction. Examples include studies showing the following:

1. Head injury and maternal alcohol intake during pregnancy are more strongly related to Performance IQ than to Verbal IQ (Chadwick et al., 1981; Streissguth et al., 1989).
2. Head injury severity is more predictably correlated with postinjury cognitive performance than with behavioral changes (Fletcher et al., 1990; Rutter, 1981).
3. Early onset diabetes and low birth weight complications are associated more closely with spatial and perceptual-motor skills than with IQ or verbal abilities (Rovet, Ehrlich, & Hoppe, 1988; Wiener et al., 1965).
4. Social factors are better predictors of IQ and achievement than of specific neuropsychological skills (Morrison & Hinshaw, 1988).
5. Maturation and schooling have differential effects on fluid versus crystallized abilities (Cahan & Cohen, 1989).

Conceiving of certain child traits as less readily modified by environmental influences than other traits also helps to explain why children with mild mental deficiency have great difficulty generalizing instruction in "thinking skills" yet can be readily taught narrowly targeted learning or adaptive strategies (Weinberg, 1989).

An important implication for studies of the effects of early brain injuries is that learning and behavior problems are not necessary consequences of early brain injuries, even in samples with obvious neuropsychological deficits (Taylor et al., 1984; Taylor, Albo, et al., 1987). Although direct evidence in this regard is lacking, supportive environments may be able to contain the effects of subtle cognitive limitations on the acquisition of academic skills and on behavioral adaptation. Unsupportive environments, on the other hand, may exacerbate the effects of brain disease, even to the point that problems in learning or behavior may be more obvious or enduring than any residual cognitive disability (Brown et al., 1981; Perrott et al., 1991). The risks that early brain injuries pose for learning and behavior therefore may be more difficult to predict, and more variable across samples, than risks for neuropsychological impairment. Inconsistencies in reports of the effects of Hib meningitis on IQ and academic achievement may well be due to such variability.

A fundamental limitation of all studies in this area to date is their failure to attempt to come to grips with the complexities of social influences on outcomes. The present investigation addressed this need by including measures of recent life events and family environment. A more complete assessment of social influences would have involved evaluation of parent adjustment, the impact of the acute-phase disease on the family and on parent–child interactions, the appropriateness of the child's management at home and school, and the resources and coping strategies employed in dealing with past or present developmental problems (Rutter, 1985). According to Masten and Garmezy, "Adaptation is an ongoing process of interactions between the systems of individual, family, social network, community, and society" (1985, pp. 36–37). Although it may be impractical to investigate social processes as comprehensively as one would like, attention to a wider array of these variables will be necessary for a more complete understanding of how early brain injuries affect development.

It is also advantageous to follow children prospectively from disease onset. The reasons for this are that prospective follow-up avoids sampling problems and provides an opportunity to trace the natural history of sequelae. The type of retrospective recruitment that characterized the present project, wherein subjects were evaluated an average of 8 years after their disease, prevents study of immediate disease consequences and of factors in the postinjury environment that either help the child to compensate or precipitate further problems. A further virtue of prospective data collection is that the investigator is in a better position to obtain information on premorbid functioning and to assess disease variables that might not otherwise be available.

As illustrated in the present study, investigation of within-sample differences is additionally warranted. Depending on sample composition, group findings may obscure the true effects of the disease; hence a search for "outliers" is recommended (Masten & Garmezy, 1985; Rutter, 1982). The child's acute-phase neurological status may be especially useful in targeting those individuals most likely to experience sequelae. As noted earlier, efforts to document neuropathological changes hold considerable promise in identifying meaningful subsets within a given sample and in exploring mechanisms of recovery (Fletcher & Levin, 1988; Landry, Chapieski, Fletcher, & Denson, 1988). The more that is known about the status of the brain and about environmental influences on outcomes, the more possible it will be to test competing hypotheses as to how sparing takes place—whether by virtue of behavioral substitution, vicarious neural functioning, or the absence of residual pathology (St. James-Roberts, 1979; Taylor, 1984). Other benefits of focusing on individual cases are the clues they provide regarding compensatory or "protective" factors (Chess, 1978; Kopp, 1983; Masten & Garmezy, 1985). Likely examples of compensation are the children in this study who manifested neuropsychological impairments and who performed far below their siblings in IQ, but who nevertheless had many age-appropriate academic skills.

Another need in designing future studies is improved measurement and statistical methodology. Major strengths of the current study were the control that was achieved over social and family background factors, the use of a comprehensive battery of age-standardized measures of outcome, a conceptual framework for posing research questions, and an analytic plan that allowed multiple tests of the hypotheses while minimizing the chances of spurious findings. One drawback was that only a minority of the sample exhibited measurable sequelae, suggesting that further work in this area will require expanded sample size or recruitment that is more selective of high-risk groups. A larger sample size also would have allowed application of structural equation modeling (Francis, 1988). The primary virtues of this method are that it encourages the development of measurement models for predictor and outcomes variables and it permits examination of the effects of early brain disease in relation to other developmental influences. Another shortcoming was that assessments of outcome were too limited. Expanded assessments might entail direct classroom observations, more extensive teacher ratings of educational progress, and evaluations of socialization, self-esteem, and personality characteristics. Progress also has been stalled by lack of uniformity in evaluation procedures, diagnostic criteria, and statistical approaches (Costa, 1988; Costello, 1989b).

Finally, neuropsychological testing could be improved as well. Further efforts are required to establish the reliability, construct validity, and normative expectations for neuropsychological tests and to develop new procedures for assessing theoretically relevant information processing skills (Brown, Rourke, & Cicchetti, 1989; Rourke, 1988; Taylor, 1989; Taylor & Fletcher, in press). A better understanding of the effects of early brain injuries on child development demands efforts to overcome each of these obstacles. The benefits of these efforts will be a more sophisticated appreciation of brain–behavior relationships in children and more effective methods for identifying and managing individual children.

Acknowledgments. This research was supported by NIH Grant HD20641, Neuropsychological Sequelae of *Haemophilus Influenzae* Meningitis, from the National Institute of Child Health and Human Development. Special appreciation is extended to project coordinators Debra Lean, Ph.D., Lilli Kormos, Ph.D., Joy Sheppard, Valerie Barsky, and Terese LaBerge. We also wish to acknowledge the collaboration of Drs. Richard Michaels, Elaine L. Mills, Gordon V. Watters, Antonio Ciampi, Ronald Gold, and Noni MacDonald.

References

Achenbach, T., & Edelbrock, C. (1983). *Manual for the Child Behavior Checklist and Revised Child Behavior Profile*. Burlington: University of Vermont.

Alajouanine, T., & Lhermitte, F. (1965). Acquired aphasia in children. *Brain*, *88*, 653–662.

Alon, U., Naveh, Y., Gardos, M., & Friedman, A. (1979). Neurological sequelae of septic meningitis: A follow-up study of 65 children. *Israel Journal of Medical Science*, *15*, 512–517.

Angoff, W. (1988). The nature–nuture debate, aptitudes, and group differences. *American Psychologist*, *43*, 713–720.

Annett, M. (1973). Laterality of children hemiplegia and the growth of speech and intelligence. *Cortex*, *9*, 4–33.

Aram, D. (1988). Language sequelae of unilateral brain lesions in children. In F. Plum (Ed.), *Language communication and the brain* (pp. 171–197). New York: Plenum.

Aram, D., & Ekelman, B. (1986). Cognitive profiles of children with early onset unilateral lesions. *Developmental Neuropsychology*, *2*, 155–172.

Aram, D., & Ekelman, B. (1988). Scholastic aptitude and achievement among children with unilateral brain lesions. *Neuropsychology*, *26*, 903–916.

Baker, L., & Decker, S. D. J. (1984). Cognitive abilities in reading-disabled children: A longitudinal study. *Journal of Child Psychology and Psychiatry*, *25*, 111–117.

Baltes, P. (1968). Longitudinal and cross-sectional sequences in the study of age and generation effects. *Human Development*, *11*, 145–171.

Banich, M., Levine, S., Kim, H., & Huttenlocher, P. (1990). The effects of developmental factors on IQ in hemiplegic children. *Neuropsychologia*, *28*, 35–47.

Bawden, H., Knights, R., & Winogron, H. W. (1985). Speeded performance following head injury in children. *Journal of Clinical and Experimental Neuropsychology*, *7*, 39–54.

Belmont, L., & Marolla, F. (1973). Birth order, family size, and intelligence. *Science*, *182*, 1096–1101.

Benton, A. (1962). Behavioral indices of brain injury in school children. *Child Development*, *33*, 199–208.

Byers, R., & Lord, E. (1943). Late effects of lead poisoning on mental development. *American Journal of Diseases of Children*, *66*, 471–494.

Byers, R., & McLean, W. (1962). Etiology and course of certain hemiplegias with aphasia in childhood. *Pediatrics*, *29*, 376–383.

Birch, H. (1964). The problem of "brain damage" in children. In H. Birch (Ed.), *Brain damage in children: The biological and social aspects* (pp. 3–12). Baltimore: William & Wilkins.

Birch, H. (1981). Neuropsychological aspects of brain dysfunction in children. In P. Black (Ed.), *Brain dysfunction in children: Etiology, diagnosis, and management* (pp. 193–201). New York: Raven Press.

Birch, H., & Bortner, M. (1967). Stimulus competition and concept utilization in brain damaged children. *Developmental Medicine and Child Neurology*, *9*, 402–410.

Bock, R. (1975). *Multivariate statistics for the behavioral sciences*. New York: McGraw-Hill.

Boll, T., & Barth, J. (1981). Neuropsychology of brain damage in children. In S. Filskov & T. Boll (Eds.), *Handbook of clinical neuropsychology* (pp. 415–452). New York: Wiley.

Borkowski, W. J., Goldgar, D., Gorga, M., Brookhouser, P., & Worthington, D. (1985). Cerebrospinal fluid parameters and auditory brainstem responses following meningitis. *Pediatric Neurology*, *1*, 134–139.

Bradley, R., Caldwell, B., & Rock, S. (1989). Home environment and cognitive development in the first 3 years of life: A collaborative study involving six sites, and three ethnic groups in North America. *Developmental Psychology*, *25*, 217–235.

Bray, J., & Maxwell, S. (1982). Analyzing and interpreting significant MANOVA's. *Review of Educational Research*, *52*, 340–367.

Breslau, N. (1983). The psychological study of chronically ill and disabled children: Are healthy siblings appropriate controls? *Journal of Abnormal Child Psychology*, *3*, 379–391.

Breslau, N. (1985). Psychiatric disorder in children with physical disability. *Journal of the American Academy of Child Psychiatry*, *24*, 87–94.

Breslau, N. (1990). Does brain dysfunction increase children's vulnerability to environmental stress. *Archives of General Psychiatry*, *47*, 15–20.

Breslau, N., Klein, N., & Allen, L. (1988). Very low brithweight: Behavioral sequelae at nine years of age. *Journal of the American Academy of Child and Adolescent Psychiatry*, *27*, 605–612.

Breslau, N., & Marshall, I. (1985). Psychological disturbance in children with physical disability: Continuity and change in a 5 year follow-up. *Journal of Abnormal Child Psychology*, *13*, 199–216.

Breslau, N., Staruch, K., & Mortimer, E. (1982). Psychological distress in mothers of disabled children. *American Journal of Diseases of Childhood*, *136*, 682–686.

Broman, S., Nichols, P., & Kennedy, W. (1975). *Preschool IQ: Prenatal and early developmental correlates*. Hillsdale, NJ: Erlbaum.

Brown, G., Chadwick, O., Shaffer, P., Rutter, M., & Traub, M. (1981). A prospective study of children with head injuries: III. Psychiatric sequelae. *Psychological Medicine*, *11*, 63–78.

Brown, S., Rourke, B., & Cicchetti, D. (1989). Reliability of tests and measures used in the neuropsychological assessment of children. *The Clinical Neuropsychologist*, *3*, 353–368.

Bryk, A., & Raudenbush, S. (1987). Application of hierarchical linear models to assessing change. *Psychological Bulletin*, *101*, 147–158.

Cahan, S., & Cohen, N. (1989). Age verses schooling effects on intelligence development. *Child Development*, *60*, 1239–1249.

Cattell, R. (1963). Theory of fluid and crystallized intelligence: A critical experiment. *Journal of Educational Psychology*, *54*, 1–22.

Chadwick, O., Rutter, M., Brown, G., Shaffer, D., & Traub, M. (1981). A prospective study of children with head injuries: II. Cognitive sequelae. *Psychological Medicine*, *11*, 49–61.

Chelune, G., & Edwards, P. (1981). Early brain lesions: Ontogenetic-environmental considerations. *Journal of Consulting and Clinical Psychology*, *49*, 777–790.

Chess, S. (1978). The plasticity of human development: Alternative pathways. *Journal of Child Psychiatry*, *17*, 80–91.

Cohen, J., & Cohen, P. (1983). *Applied multiple regression/correlational analysis for the behavioral sciences*. Hillsdale, NJ: Erlbaum.

Cohen, S. (1986). The low birthweight infant and learning disabilities. In M. Lewis (Ed.), *Learning disabilities and prenatal risk* (pp. 153–193). Urbana: University of Illinois Press.

Costa, L. (1988). Clinical neuropsychology: Prospects and problems. *The Clinical Neuropsychologist*, *2*, 3–11.

Costello, E. J. (1989a). Child psychiatric disorders and their correlates: A primary care pediatric sample. *Journal of the American Academy of Child and Adolescent Psychiatry*, *28*, 851–855.

Costello, E. J. (1989b). Developments in child psychiatric epidemiology. *Journal of the American Academy of Child and Adolescent Psychiatry*, *28*, 836–841.

Coulehan, J., Michaels, R., Williams, K. L. D., North, Q., Welty, T., & Rogers, K. (1976). Bacterial meningitis in Navajo Indians. *Public Health Reports*, *91*, 464–468.

Crnic, K., Friedrich, W., & Greenberg, M. (1983). Adaptation of families with mentally retarded children: A model of stress, coping, and family ecology. *American Journal of Mental Deficiency*, *88*, 125–138.

Crnic, K., Grenberg, M., Ragozin, A., Robinson, N., & Basham, R. (1983). Effects of stress and social support on mothers and premature and full-term infants. *Child Development*, *54*, 209–217.

Crnic, K., Ragozin, A., Greenberg, M., Robinson, N., & Basham, R. (1983). Social interaction and developmental competence of preterm and full-term infants during the first year of life. *Child Development*, *54*, 1199–1210.

Crothers, B., & Lord, E. (1938). Appraisal of intellectual and physical factors after cerebral damage in children. *American Journal of Psychiatry*, *94*, 1077–1080.

Cullinan, D., Epstein, M., & Lloyd, J. (1981). School behavior problems of learning disabled and normal girls and boys. *Learning Disabilities Quarterly*, *4*, 163–169.

Davidson, P., Willoughby, R., O'Luam, L., Swisher, C., & Benjamins, P. (1978). Neurological and intellectual sequelae of Reye's syndrome. *American Journal of Mental Deficiency*, *82*, 535–541.

Davie, R., Butler, N., & Goldstein, H. (1972). *From birth to seven: A report of the National Child Development Study*. London: Logman.

Davies, P. (1989). Long-term effects of meningitis. *Developmental Medicine and Child Neurology*, *31*, 398–400.

Decker, S., & DeFries, J. (1981). Cognitive ability profiles in families of reading-disabled children. *Developmental Medicine Child Neurology*, *23*, 217–227.

Dennis, M. (1974). Selective impairments of visuo-spatial abilities in infantile hemiplegia after right cerebral hemidecortication. *Neuropsychology*, *12*, 505–512.

Dennis, M. (1980). Capacity and strategy for syntactic comprehension after left or right hemidecortication. *Brain and Language*, *10*, 287–317.

Dennis, M., Fitz, C. R., Netley, C. T., Sugar, J., Harwood-Nash, D. C. F., Hendricks, E. B., Hoffman, H. J., & Humphreys, R. P. (1981). The intelligence of hydrocephalic children. *Archives of Neurology*, *38*, 607–615.

Dennis, M., Hendrick, E., Hoffman, H., & Humphreys, R. (1987). Language of hydrocephalic children and adolescents. *Journal of Clinical and Experimental Neuropsychology*, *9*, 593–621.

Dennis, M., & Whitaker, H. (1976). Language acquisition following hemidecortication: Linguistic superiority of the left over the right hemisphere. *Brain and Language*, *3*, 404–433.

Dikmen, S., Matthews, C., & Harley, J. (1975). The effect of early vs late onset of major motor epilepsy upon cognitive-intellectual performance. *Epilepsy*, *16*, 73–81.

Dodge, P. (1986). Sequelae of bacterial meningitis. *Pediatric Infectious Disease*, *5*, 618–620.

Dodge, P., Davis, H., & Feigin, R., Holmes, S. J., Kaplan, S. L., Jubelirer, D. P., Stechenberg, B. W., & Hirsh, S. K. (1984). Prospective evaluation of hearing impairment as a sequela of acute bacterial meningitis. *New England Journal of Medicine*, *311*, 869–874.

Dodge, P., & Swartz, M. (1965). Bacterial meningitis: A review of selected aspects: II. Special neurologic problems, postmeningitis complications and clinicopathological correlations. *New England Journal of Medicine*, *272*, 954–960, 1003–1010.

Drillien, C., Thomson, A., & Burgoyne, K. (1980). Low birthweight children at early school age: A longitudinal study. *Developmental Medicine and Child Neurology*, *22*, 25–47.

Earls, F. (1987). Sex differences in psychiatric disorders: Origins and developmental influences. *Psychiatric Development*, *1*, 1–23.

Emmett, M., Jeffery, H., Chandler, D., & Dugdale, A. (1980). Sequelae of *Hemophilus influenzae* meningitis. *Australian Paediatric Journal*, *16*, 90–93.

Escalona, S. (1982). Babies at double hazard: Early development of infants at biologic and social risks. *Pediatrics*, *70*, 670–676.

Escalona, S. (1984). Social and other environmental influences on the cognitive and personality developmental of low birth weight infants. *American Journal of Mental Deficiency*, *88*, 508–512.

Eskola, J., Peltola, H., Takala, A., Kayhty, H., Hakulinen, M., Karanko, V., Kela, E., Rekola, P., Ronnberg, P. R., Samuelson, J. S., Gordon, L. K., & Makela, P. H. (1987). Efficacy of *Haemophilus influenzae* type b polysaccharide-diphtheria toxoid conjugate vaccine in infancy. *New England Journal of Medicine*, *317*, 717–722.

Estes, W. (1981). Intelligence and learning. In M. P. Friedman, J. P. Das, & N. O'Connor (Eds.), *Intelligence and learning* (pp. 3–23). New York: Plenum.

Ewing-Cobbs, L., Fletcher, J., & Levin, H. (1985). Neuropsychological sequelae following pediatric head injury. In M. Ylvisaker (Ed.), *Head injury rehabilitation* (pp. 71–90). San Diego: College-Hill.

Ewing-Cobbs, L., Levin, H., Eisenberg, H., & Fletcher, J. (1987). Language disorders after pediatric head injury in children. *Journal of Clinical and Experimental Neuropsychology*, *9*, 575–592.

Feigin, R., Stechenberg, B., Chang, M., Dunkle, L. M., Wong, M. L., Palkes, H., Dodge, P. R., & Davis, H. (1976). Prospective evaluation of treatment of *Hemophilus influenzae* meningitis. *Journal of Pediatrics*, *88*, 542–548.

Feldman, H., & Michaels, R. (1988). Academic achievement in children 10 to 12 year after *Haemophilus influenzae* meningitis. *Pediatrics*, *81*, 339–344.

Feldman, W., Ginsburg, C., McCracken, G. J., Jr., Allen, D., Ahmann, P., Graham, J., & Graham, L. (1982). Relation of concentrations of *Haemophilus influenzae* type b in cerebrospinal fluid to late sequelae of patients with meningitis. *Journal of Pediatrics*, *100*, 209–212.

Ferry, P., Culbertson, J., Cooper, J., Sitton, A., & Sell, S. (1982). Sequelae of *Hemophilus influenzae* meningitis: Preliminary report of a long-term follow-up study. In S. Sell & P. Wright (Eds.), *Haemophilus influenzae: Epidemiology, immunology, and prevention of disease* (pp. 111–117). New York: Elsevier Biomedical.

Field, T. (1983). Social interactions between high-risk infants and their mothers, fathers, and grandmothers. In B. Lahey & A. Kazdin (Eds.), *Advances in clinical child psychology* (Vol. 6, pp. 251–283). New York: Plenum.

Finger, S., LeVere, T., Almli, C., & Stein, D. (1988). Recovery of function: Sources of controversy. In S. Finger, T. LeVere, C. Almli, & D. Stein (Eds.), *Brain injury and recovery: Theoretical and controversial issues* (pp. 351–361). New York: Plenum.

Finlayson, M., Johnson, K., & Reitan, R. (1977). Relationship of level of education to neuropsychological measures in brain-damaged and non–brain-damaged adults. *Journal of Consulting and Clinical Psychology*, *45*, 536–542.

Fletcher, J., & Copeland, D. (1988). Neurobehavioral effects of central nervous system prophylactic treatment of cancer in children. *Journal of Clinical and Experimental Neuropsychology*, *10*, 495–538.

Fletcher, J., Ewing-Cobbs, L., Miner, M., Levin, H., & Eisenberg, H. (1990). Behavioral changes after closed head injury in children. *Journal of Consulting and Clinical Psychology*, *58*, 93–98.

Fletcher, J., & Levin, H. (1988). Neurobehavioral effects of brain injury in children. In D. K. Routh (Ed.), *Handbook of pediatric psychology* (pp. 258–298). New York: Guilford.

Fletcher, J., Levin, J., & Landry, S. (1984). Behavioral consequences of cerebral insult in infancy. In C. Almli & S. Finger, (Ed.), *Early brain damage: Research orientation and clinical observations* (pp. 189–211). Orlando, FL: Academic Press.

Francis, D. (1988). An introduction to structural equation models. *Journal of Clinical and Experimental Neuropsychology*, *10*, 623–639.

Francis, D., Fletcher, J., Maxwell, S., & Satz, P. (1989). A structural model for developmental changes in the determinants of reading achievement. *Journal of Clinical Child Psychology*, *18*, 44–51.

Fraser, D. (1982). *Haemophilus influenzae* in the community and the home. In S. H. Sell & P. F. Wright (Eds.), *Haemophilus influenzae: Epidemiology, immunology, and prevention of disease* (pp. 11–24). New York: Elsevier Biomedical.

Fuld, P., & Fisher P. (1977). Recovery of intellectual ability after closed head injury. *Developmental Medicine and Child Neurology*, *19*, 495–502.

Garmezy, N., Masten, A., & Tellegen, A. (1984). The study of stress and competence in children: A building block for developmental psychopathology. *Child Development*, *55*, 97–111.

Garmezy, N., Tellegen, A., & Dervine, V. (1981). *Project competence: Studies of stress-resistant children*. Minneapolis: University of Minnesota Press.

Goldman, P. (1974). An alternative to developmental plasticity: Heterology of CNS structures in infants and adults. In P. G. Stein, J. J. Rosen, & N. Butlers (Eds.), *Plasticity and recovery of function in the central nervous system* (pp. 149–174). New York: Academic Press.

Goldman, P., & Lewis, M. (1978). Developmental biology of brain damage and experience. In C. Cotman (Ed.), *Neural plasticity* (pp. 291–310). New York: Raven Press.

Green, J. A. (1988). Loglinear analysis of cross-classified ordinal data: Applications in developmental research. *Child Development*, *59*, 1–25.

Greenberg, M., & Crnic, K. (1988). Longitudinal predictors of developmental status and social interaction in premature and full-term infants at age two. *Child Development*, *59*, 554–570.

Hack, M., & Breslau, N. (1986). Effects of brain growth in infancy on 3 year IQ in very low birthweight infants. *Pediatrics*, *77*, 196–202.

Hakuta, K. (1987). Degree of bilingualism and cognitive ability in mainland Puerto Rican children. *Child Development*, *58*, 1372–1388.

Headings, D., & Glasgow, L. (1977). Occlusion on the internal carotid artery complicating *Haemophilus influenzae* meningitis. *American Journal of Diseases of Childhood*, *131*, 854–856.

Hebb, D. (1942). The effect of early and late brain injury upon test scores, and the nature of normal adult intelligence. *Proceedings of the American Philosophical Society*, *85*, 265–292.

Hebb, D. (1949). *The organization of behavior*. New York: Wiley.

Hebb, D., & Morton, M. (1944). Note on the measurement of adult intelligence. *Journal of General Psychology*, *30*, 217–223.

Hecaen, H. (1976). Acquired aphasia in children and the ontogenesis of hemispheric functional specialization. *Brain*, *3*, 114–134.

Herson, V., & Todd, J. (1977). Prediction of morbidity in *Hemophilus influenzae* meningitis. *Pediatrics*, *59*, 35–39.

Hollingshead, A. (1957). *Two-factor index of social position*. New Haven: Yale University Press.

Horn, J. (1968). Organization of abilities and the development of intelligence. *Psychological Review*, *75*, 242–259.

Huberty, C., & Morris, J. (1989). Multivariate analysis versus multiple univariate analyses. *Psychological Bulletin*, *105*, 302–308.

Jadavji, T., Biggar, W., Gold, R., & Prober, C. (1986). Sequelae of acute bacterial meningitis in children treated for seven days. *Pediatrics*, *78*, 21–25.

Jones, F., & Hanson, D. (1977). *H. influenzae* meningitis treated with ampicillin or chloramphenicol, and subsequent hearing loss. *Developmental Medicine and Child Neurology*, *19*, 593–597.

Kaplan, S., Catlin, R. I., Weaver, T., & Feigin, R. D. (1984). Onset of hearing loss in children with bacterial meningitis. *Pediatrics*, *73*, 575–578.

Kaplan, S., Smith, E., Wills, C., & Feigin, R. (1986). Association between preadmission oral antibiotic therapy and cerebrospinal fluid findings and sequelae caused by *Haemophilus influenzae* type b. *Pediatric Infectious Disease*, *5*, 626.

Kindlon, D., Sollee, N., & Yondo, R. (1988). Specificity of behavior problems among children with neurological dysfunctions. *Journal of Pediatric Psychology*, *13*, 39–47.

Klein, J., Feigin, R., & McCracken, G. J (1986). Report of the task force on diagnosis and management of meningitis. *Pediatrics*, *78*, 959–982.

Klein, N., Hack, M., & Breslau, N. (1989). Children who were very low birthweight: Developmental and academic achievement at nine years of age. *Developmental and Behavioral Pediatrics*, *10*, 32–37.

Klonoff, H., & Low, M. (1974). Disordered brain function in young children and early adolescents: Neuropsychological and electroencephalographic correlates. In R. Reitan & L. Davison (Eds.), *Clinical neuropsychology: Current status and applications* (pp. 121–178). New York: John Wiley and Sons.

Klonoff, H., Low, M., & Clark, C. (1977). Head injuries in children: A prospective 5-year follow-up. *Journal of Neurology, Neurosurgery and Psychiatry*, *40*, 1211–1219.

Kohn, B., & Dennis, M. (1974). Somatosensory functions after cerebral hemidecortication for infantile hemiplegia. *Neuropsychology*, *12*, 119–130.

Kolb, B. (1989). Brain development, plasticity, and behavior. *American Psychologist*, *44*, 1203–1212.

Kopp, C. (1983). Risk factors in development. In M. M. Haith & J. J. Campos (Eds.), *Handbook of child psychology: Infancy and developmental psychology* (Vol. 2, pp. 1081–1188). New York: Wiley.

Kopp, C., & Krakow, J. (1983). The developmentalist and the study of biological risk: A view of the past with an eye toward the future. *Child Development*, *5*, 1086–1088.

Kresky, B., Buchbinder, S., & Greenberg, I. (1962). The incidence of neurologic residua in children after recovery from bacterial meningitis. *Archives of Pediatrics*, *79*, 63–71.

Laing, J., & Sines, J. (1981). *The Home Environment Questionnaire: An instrument for assessing several behaviorally relevant dimensions of children's environment*. Department of Psychology, University of Iowa.

Landry, S., Chapieski, L., Fletcher, J., & Denson, S. (1988). Three-year outcomes for low birth weight infants: Differential effects of early medical complications. *Journal of Pediatric Psychology*, *13*, 317–327.

Lansdell, H. (1969). Verbal and non-verbal factors in right hemisphere speech: Relation to early neurological history. *Journal of Comparative and Physiological Psychology*, *69*, 734–738.

Laurence, S., & Stein, D. (1978). Recovery after brain damage and the concept of localization of function. In S. Finger (Ed.), *Recovery from brain damage: Research and theory* (pp. 369–409). New York: Plenum.

Lebel, M. H., Freij, B. J., Syrogiannopoulos, G. A., Chrane, D. F., Hoyt, M. J., Stewart, S., Kennard, B. D., Olsen, K. D., & McCracken, G. H., Jr. (1988). Dexamethasone therapy for bacterial meningitis: Results of two double-blind placebo-controlled trials. *New England Journal of Medicine*, *319*, 964–971.

Lenneberg, E. (1967). *Biological foundations of language*. New York: Wiley.

Levin, H., & Eisenberg, H. (1979). Neuropsychological outcome of closed head injury in children and adolescents. *Child's Brain*, *5*, 281–292.

Levin, H., Eisenberg, H., Wiig, N., & Kobayaski, K. (1982). Memory and intellectual ability after head injury in children and adolescents. *Neurosurgery*, *11*, 668–672.

Levin, H., Ewing-Cobbs, L., & Benton, A. (1987). Age and recovery from brain damage: A review of clinical studies. In S. Scheff (Ed.), *Aging and recovery of function* (pp. 169–204). New York: Plenum.

Lewin, R. (1980). Is your brain necessary? *Science*, *210*, 1232–1234.

Lindberg, J., Rosenhall, U., Nylen, O., & Ringner, A. (1977). Long-term outcome of *Hemophilus influenzae* meningitis related to antibiotic treatment. *Pediatrics*, *60*, 1–6.

Lord, E. (1937). *Children handicapped by cerebral palsy: Psychological factors in management*. London: Commonwealth Fund Books; New York: Oxford University Press.

MacDonald, J., & Feinstein, S. (1984). Hearing loss following *Hemophilus influenzae* meningitis in infancy. *Archives of Neurology*, *41*, 1058–1059.

Mash, E., & Barkley, R. (1989). *Treatment of childhood disorders*. New York: Guilford Press.

Masten, A. S., & Garmezy, N. (1985). Risk, vulnerability, and protective factors in developmental psychopathology. In B. Lahey & A. Kazdin (Eds.), *Advances in clinical child psychology* (Vol. 9, pp. 1–52). New York: Plenum.

McConaughy, S., & Achenbach, T. (1988). *Practical guide for the Child Behavior Checklist and related materials*. Department of Psychiatry, University of Vermont.

McNemar, Q. (1969). *Psychological statistics*. New York: Wiley.

Michaels, R., & Schultz, W. (1973). The frequency of *Hemophilus influenzae* infections: Analysis of racial and environmental factors. In S. Sell & D. Rarzon (Eds.), *Hemophilus influenzae: Proceedings of a conference on antigen–antibody systems, epidemiology, and immunoprophylaxis* (pp. 243–250). Nashville: Vanderbilt University Press.

Mills, E., MacDonald, N., Gold, R., & Taylor, H. (1988). *Neurodevelopmental consequences of Haemophilus influenzae meningitis*. Paper presented at the meeting of the Society for Pediatric Research, Washington, DC.

Morrison, D., & Hinshaw, S. (1988). The relationship between neuropsychological/perceptual performance and socioeconomic status in children with learning disabilities. *Journal of Learning Disabilities*, *21*, 124–128.

Myer, E., & Byers, R. (1952). Measles encephalitis. *American Journal of Diseases of Childhood*, *84*, 853–879.

Nelson, H. A. (1980). Longitudinal study of the psychological aspect of myelomenigocele. *Scandinavian Journal of Psychology*, *21*, 45–54.

Nichols, P., & Chen, T. (1981). *Minimal brain dysfunction: A prospective study*. Hillsdale, NJ: Erlbaum.

Nussbaum, N., Grant, M., Roman, M., Poole, J., & Bigler, E. (1990). Attention deficit disorder and the mediating effect of age on academic and behavioral variables. *Developmental and Behavioral Pediatrics*, *11*, 22–26.

O'Brien, R., & Kaiser, M. (1985). MANOVA method for analyzing repeated measures designs: An extensive primer. *Psychological Bulletin*, *97*, 316–333.

O'Dougherty, M., Wright, F., Garmezy, N., Loewenson, R., & Torres, F. (1983). Later competence and adaptation in infants who survive severe heart defects. *Child Development 54*, 1129–1942.

O'Leary, P., & Seidenberg, M. (1981). Effects of age of onset of tonic-clonic seizure on neuropsychological performance in children. *Epilepsy*, *22*, 197–204.

Olweus, D., Block, J., & Radke-Yarrow, M. (1986). *Development of antisocial and prosocial behavior: Research, theory, and issues*. Orlando, FL: Academic Press.

Parkinson, C., & Wallis, C. (1981). School achievement and behavior of children small for dates at birth. *Developmental Medicine and Child Neurology*, *28*, 41–50.

Parkinson, C., Wallis, C., & Harvey, D. (1981). School achievement and behavior in children small for dates at birth. *Developmental Medicine and Child Neurology*, *28*, 41–50.

Pasamanick, B., & Knobloch, H. (1961). Syndrome of minimal cerebral damage in infancy. *Journal of the American Medical Association*, *170*, 1384–1387.

Peloquin, L., & Davidson, P. (1989). Psychological sequelae of pediatric infectious diseases. In D. Routh (Ed.), *Handbook of pediatric psychology* (pp. 222–257). New York: Guilford Press.

Perrott, S., Taylor, H., & Montes, J. (1991). Neuropsychological sequelae, familial stress, and environmental adaption following pediatric head injury. *Developmental Neuropsychology*, *7*(1), 69–86.

Piercy, M. (1964). The effects of cerebral lesions on intellectual functions: A review of current research trends. *British Journal of Psychiatry*, *110*, 310–322.

Plomin, R. (1989). Environment and genes: Determinants of behavior. *American Psychologist*, *44*, 105–111.

Rasmussen, T., & Milner, B. (1977). The role of early left-brain injury in determining lateralization of cerebral speech functions. *Annals of the New York Academy of Sciences*, *299*, 355–369.

Reitan, R. (1974). Psychological effects of cerebral lesions in children of early school age. In R. Reitan & L. Davison (Ed.), *Clinical neuropsychology: Current status and applications* (pp. 53–89). New York: Wiley.

Reynolds, C. (1981). The neuropsychological basis of intelligence. In G. Hynd & J. Obrzut (Ed.), *Neuropsychological assessment of the school-aged child: Issues and procedures* (pp. 87–124). New York: Grune & Stratton.

Rogosa, D., Brandt, D., & Zimowski, M. (1982). A growth curve approach to the measurement of change. *Psychological Bulletin*, *92*, 726–748.

Rosenhall, U., Nylen, O., Lindberg, J., & Kankkunen, A. (1978). Auditory function after *Haemophilus influenzae* meningitis. *Acta Otolaryngology*, *85*, 243–247.

Rourke, B. (1982). Central processing deficiencies in children: Toward a developmental neuropsychological model. *Journal of Clinical Neuropsychology*, *4*, 1–18.

Rourke, B. (1988). The syndrome of nonverbal learning disabilities: Developmental manifestations in neurological disease, disorder, and dysfunction. *Clinical Neuropsychologist*, *2*, 293–330.

Rourke, B., Bakker, D., Fisk, J., & Strang, J. (1983). *Child neuropsychology: Introduction to theory, research and clinical practice*. New York: Guilford Press.

Rourke, B., Fisk, J., & Strang, J. (1986). *Neuropsychological assessment of children: A treatment approach*. New York: Guilford Press.

Rovet, J., Ehrlich, R., & Hoppe, M. (1988). Specific intellectual deficits in children with early onset diabetes melitis. *Child Development*, *59*, 226–234.

Rudel, R., Teuber, H., & Twitchell, T. (1974). Levels of impairment of sensorimotor function in children with early brain damage. *Neuropsychologia*, *12*, 95–108.

Russell, W. (1948). Functions of the frontal lobes. *Lancet*, *1*, 356–360.

Rutter, M. (1977). Brain damage syndromes in children: Concepts and findings. *Journal of Child Psychology and Psychiatry*, *18*, 1–21.

Rutter, M. (1981). Psychological sequelae of brain damage in children. *American Journal of Psychiatry*, *138*, 1533–1544.

Rutter, M. (1982). Developmental neuropsychiatry: Concepts, issues, and problems. *Journal of Clinical Neuropsychiatry*, *4*, 91–115.

Rutter, M. (1985). Family and school influences on behavioral development. *Journal of Child Psychology and Psychiatry*, *26*, 349–368.

Rutter, M., Chadwick, O., Shaffer, D., & Brown, G. (1980). A prospective study of children with head injuries: I. Design and methods. *Psychological Medicine*, *10*, 633–645.

Rutter, M., Graham, P., & Yule, W. (1970). A neuropsychiatric study in childhood. *Clinics in developmental medicine* (pp. 35–36). London: Heinemann Medical Books.

Ryan, C., Morrow, L., Bromet, E., & Parkinson, D. (1987). Assessment of neuropsychological dysfunction in the workplace: Normative data from the Pittsburgh occupational exposures test battery. *Journal of Clinical and Experimental Neuropsychology*, *9*, 665–679.

Sameroff, A., & Chandler, M. (1975). Reproductive risk and the continuum of caretaking casualty. In F. Horowitz (Ed.), *Review of child development research* (pp. 187–244). Chicago: University of Chicago Press.

Satz, P. (1987, June). *Developmental dyslexia: An etiological reformulation*. Paper presented at Third World Congress of Dyslexia. Crete, Greece.

Satz, P., & Bullard-Bates, C. (1981). Acquired aphasia in children. In M. Sarno (Ed.), *Acquired aphasia* (pp. 399–426). New York: Academic Press.

Schaad, U., Suter, S., Gianella-Borradori, A., Pfenninger, J., Auckenthaler, R., Bernath, O., Cheseaux, J. J., & Wedgewood, J. (1990). A comparison of ceftriaxone and cefuroxime for treatment of bacterial meningitis in children. *New England Journal of Medicine*, *322*, 141–147.

Schneider, G. E. (1979). Is it really better to have your brain early: A revision of the "Kennard Principal." *Neuropsychologia*, *17*, 557–583.

Schonfeld, I., Shaffer, D., O'Connor, P., & Portnoy, S. (1988). Conduct disorder and cognitive functioning: Testing three causal hypotheses. *Child Development*, *59*, 993–1007.

Seidel, U., Chadwick, O., & Rutter, M. (1975). Psychological disorders in crippled children: A comparative study of children with and without brain damage. *Developmental Medicine and Child Neurology*, *17*, 563–573.

Sell, F. (1986). Outcome of very low birthweight infants. *Clinics in Perinatology*, *12*, 451–459.

Sell, S. (1983). Long term sequelae of bacterial meningitis in children. *Pediatric Infectious Disease*, *2*, 90–93.

Sell, S., Merrill, R., Doyne, E., & Zimsky, E., Jr. (1972). Long-term sequelae of *Hemophilus influenzae* meningitis. *Pediatrics*, *49*, 206–211.

Sell, S., Webb, W., Pate, J., & Doyne, E. (1972). Psychological sequelae to bacterial meningitis: Two controlled studies. *Pediatrics*, *49*, 212–217.

Shaffer, D. (1985). Brain damage. In M. Rutter & L. Hersov (Eds.), *Child and adolescent psychiatry* (pp. 129–151). Boston: Blackwell Scientific.

Siegel, L. (1981). Infant tests as predictors of cognitive and language development at two years. *Child Development*, *52*, 545–557.

Sigman, M., & Parmalee, A. H. (1979). Longitudinal evaluation of the preterm infant. In T. Field, A. Sostek, S. Goldberg, & H. Shuman (Eds.), *Infants born at risk: Behavior and development* (pp. 271–296). New York: Spectrum.

Sines, J. (1987). Influence of the home and family environment on childhood dysfunction. In B. Lahey & A. Kazdin (Eds.), *Advances in clinical child psychology* (Vol. 10, pp. 1–54). New York: Plenum.

Smith, A., & Sugar, C. (1975). Development of above normal language and intelligence 21 years after left hemispherectomy. *Neurology*, *25*, 813–818.

Smith, M., Delves, T., Lansdown, R., Clayton, B., & Graham, P. (1983). The effects of lead exposure on urban children: The Institute of Child Health/ Southampton Study. *Developmental Medicine and Child Neurology*, Supplement No. 47, *25*(5), 1–38.

Snyder, R., Stovring, J., Cushing, A. Davis, L., & Hardy, T. (1981). Cerebral infarction in childhood bacterial meningitis. *Journal of Neurology, Neurosurgery, and Psychiatry*, *44*, 581–585.

Soper, H., Cicchetti, D., Satz, P., Light, R., & Orsini, D. (1988). Null hypothesis disrespect in neuropsychology: Danger of alpha and beta errors. *Journal of Clinical and Experimental Neuropsychology*, *10*, 255–270.

Sparrow, S., Bolla, D., & Cicchetti, D. (1984). *Vineland Adaptive Behavior Scales*. Circle Pines, MN: American Guidance Service.

Sproles, E., Azerrad, J., Williamson, C., & Merrill, R. (1969). Meningitis due to *Hemophilus influenzae*: Long-term sequelae. *Journal of Pediatrics*, *75*, 782–788.

St. James-Roberts, I. (1979). Neurological plasticity, recovery from brain insult and child development. In H. W. Reese & L. Lipsett (Eds.), *Advances in child development and behavior* (pp. 253–319). New York: Academic Press.

St. James-Roberts, I. (1981). A reinterpretation of hemispherectomy data without functional plasticity of the brain: Intellectual function. *Brain and Language*, *1*, 31–53.

Stoving, J., & Snyder, R. (1980). Computed tomography in childhood bacterial meningitis. *Journal of Pediatrics*, *96*, 820–823.

Streissguth, A., Barr, H., Sampson, P., Darby, B., & Martin, D. (1989). IQ at age 4 in relation to maternal alcohol use and smoking during pregnancy. *Developmental Psychology*, *25*, 3–11.

Swaiman, K., & Wright, F. (1982). *The practice of pediatric neurology*. St. Louis: Mosby.

Swartz, M. (1984). Bacterial meningitis. *New England Journal of Medicine 311*, 912–914.

Synder, R., Stovring, J., Cushing, A., Davis, L., & Hardy, T. (1981). Cerebral infarction in childhood bacterial meningitis. *Journal of Neurology, Neurosurgery, and Psychiatry*, *44*, 581–585.

Tatsuoka, M. (1971). *Multivariate analysis: Techniques for educational and psychological research*. New York: Wiley.

Taylor, E. (1959). *Psychological appraisal of children with cerebral defects*. Cambridge, MA: Harvard University Press.

Taylor, H. (1984). Early brain injury and cognitive development. In C. Almli & S. Finger (Eds.), *Early brain damage: Research orientations and clinical observations* (pp. 325–345). New York: Academic Press.

Taylor, H. (1987). Childhood sequelae of early neurological disorders: A contemporary perspective. *Developmental Neuropsychology*, *3*, 153–164.

Taylor, H. (1988). Neuropsychological testing: Relevance for assessing children's learning disabilities. *Journal of Consulting and Clinical Psychology*, *56*, 795–800.

Taylor, H., Albo, V., Phebus, C., Sachs, B., & Bierl, P. (1987). Postirradiation treatment outcomes for children with acute lymphocytic leukemia: Clarification of risks. *Journal of Pediatric Psychology*, *12*, 395–411.

Taylor, H., & Fletcher, J. (1990). Neuropsychological assessment of children. In G. Goldstein & Herson, M. (Eds.), *Handbook of psychological assessment* (2nd ed., pp. 228–255). New York: Pergamon.

Taylor, H., Lean, D., Michaels, R., & Mills, E. (1987). *Neurodevelopmental consequences of H flu meningitis in children*. Paper presented at the meeting of the American Psychological Association, New York.

Taylor, H., Michaels, R., Mazur, P., Bauer, R., & Liden, C. (1984). Intellectual, neuropsychological, and achievement outcomes in children six to eight years after recovery from *Haemophilus influenzae* meningitis. *Pediatrics*, *72*, 198–205.

Taylor, H., Mills, E., Ciampi, A., DuBerger, R., Watters, G., Gold, R., MacDonald, N., & Michaels, R. (1990). The sequelae of *Haemophilus influenzae* in school-age children. *New England Journal of Medicine*, *323*, 1657–1663.

Taylor, H., Mills, E., Watters, G., & Kormos, L. (1988, January). *The significance of neuropsychological sequelae in childhood survivors of H. flu meningitis*. Paper presented at the meeting of the International Neuropsychological Society, New Orleans, LA.

Taylor, H., & Schatschneider, C. (1989, June). *Learning problems in children who have recovered from meningitis: Evidence for biological, social, and cognitive antecedents*. Paper presented at the Conference on Learning Disabilities, Ann Arbor, MI.

Taylor, H., & Schatschneider, C. (1990, February). *The significance of neuropsychological test results in children who have recovered from meningitis*. Paper presented at International Neuropsychological Society, Orlando, FL.

Tejani, A., Dobias, B., & Samburksy, J. (1982). Long-term prognosis after *H influenzae* meningitis: Prospective evaluation. *Developmental Medicine and Child Neurology*, *24*, 338–343.

Teuber, H. (1975). Recovery of function after brain injury in man. In Ciba Foundation Symposium, *Outcome of severe damage to the central nervous system* (pp. 159–190). Amsterdam: Elsevier.

Teuber, H., & Rudel, R. (1962). Behavior after cerebral lesions in children and adults. *Developmental Medicine and Child Neurology*, *4*, 3–20.

Thomas, V., & Hopkins, I. (1972). Anteriographic demonstration of vascular lesions in the study of neurologic deficit in advanced *Haemophilus influenzae* meningitis. *Developmental Medicine and Child Neurology*, *14*, 783–787.

Thompson, L. (in press). Genetic contributions to intellectual development in infancy and childhood. In P. Vernon (Ed.), *Biological approaches to the study of human intelligence*. New York: Ablex.

Thompson, N. M., Francis, D., Fletcher, J., Ewing-Cobbs, L., Levin, H., & Miner, M. (1990, February). *Recovery of spatial, motor, and perceptual skills following closed head injury in children*. Paper presented at the International Neuropsychological Society, Orlando, FL.

Thompson, R., Kronenberger, W., Johnson, D., & Whiting, K. (1989). The role of central nervous system functioning and family functioning in behavioral problems of children with myelodysplasia. *Developmental and Behavioral Pediatrics*, *10*, 242–248.

Timm, N. (1977). *Multivariate analysis*. Monterey, CA: Books-Cole.

Van Dongen, H., & Loonen, M. (1977). Factors related to prognosis of acquired aphasia in children. *Cortex*, *13*, 131–236.

Vargha-Khadem, F., Isaacs, E., Papaleloudi, H., Polkey, C., & Wilson, J. (in press). Representational language and the isolated right hemisphere. *Brain*.

Vargha-Khadem, F., O'Gorman, A., & Watters, G. (1985). Development of speech and language following bilateral frontal lesions. *Brain and Language*, *25*, 167–183.

Vernon, P. (1981). Reaction time and intelligence in the mentally retarded. *Intelligence*, *5*, 345–355.

Vohr, B. R., & Coll, C. T. (1985). Neurodevelopmental and school performance of very low-birth-weight infants: A seven year longitudinal study. *Pediatrics*, *76*, 345–350.

Vohr, B., & Garcia-Coll, C. (1988). Follow-up studies of high-risk low-birthweight infants: Changing trends. In H. Fitzgerald, B. Lester, & M. Yogman (Eds.), *Theory and research in behavioral pediatrics* (Vol. 1, pp. 1–65). New York: Plenum.

Vygotsky, L. (1962). *Thought and language*. Cambridge, MA: MIT Press.

Waber, D., Urion, D., & Tarbell, N. (1990). Later effects of central nervous system treatment of acute lymphoblastic leukemia in childhood are sex-dependent. *Developmental Medicine and Child Neurology*, *32*, 238–248.

Wachs, T. (1982). *Early experience and human development*. New York: Plenum.

Wallander, J., Varni, J., Babani, L., Banis, H., & Wilcox, K. (1989). Family resources as resistance factors for psychological maladjustment in chronically ill and handicapped children. *Journal of Pediatric Psychology*, *14*, 157–173.

Wechsler, D. (1974). *The Wechsler Intelligence Scale for Children—Revised*. New York: Psychological Corporation.

Weinberg, R. (1989). Intelligence and IQ: Landmark issues and great debates. *American psychologist*, *44*, 98–104.

Wiener, G., Rider, R., Oppel, W., Fisher, L., & Harper, P. (1965). Correlates of low birth weight: Psychological status at six to seven years of age. *Pediatrics*, *35*, 434–444.

Werner, E., & Smith, R. (1982). *Vulnerable but invincible: A longitudinal study of resilient children and youth*. New York: McGraw-Hill.

Wills, K., Holmbeck, G., Dillon, K., & McLone, D. (1990). Intelligence and achievement in children with myelomeningocele. *Journal of Pediatric Psychology*, *15*, 161–176.

Witelson, S. (1987). Neurobiological aspects of language in children. *Child Development*, *58*, 653–688.

Wolff, P. (1981). Normal variation in human maturation. In K. Connolly & H. F. R. Prechtl (Eds.) *Clinics in developmental medicine 77, 78: Maturation and development: Biological and psychological perspectives* (pp. 1–18). London: Heinemann Medical Books.

Woods, B. (1980). The restricted effects of right hemisphere lesions after age one: Wechsler test data. *Neuropsychologia*, *18*, 65–70.

Woods, B., & Carey, S. (1979). Language deficits after apparent recovery from childhood aphasia. *Annals of Neurology*, *6*, 405–409.

Woods, B., & Teuber, H. (1978). Changing patterns of childhood aphasia. *Annals of Neurology*, *3*, 273–280.

Wright, L. (1978). A method for predicting sequelae to meningitis. *American Psychologist*, *33*, 1037–1039.

Wright, L., & Jimmerson, S. (1971). Intellectual sequelae of *Hemophilus influenzae* meningitis. *Journal of Abnormal Psychology*, *77*, 181–183.

Ylvisaker, M. (1985). *Head injury rehabilitation: Children and adolescents*. San Diego: College-Hill.

CHAPTER 4

Behavioral Disturbance in Children with Seizures

ALISON D. CURLEY

There is an increased incidence of behavioral deviance among children with seizures (Trimble & Cull, 1988). This has been the subject of research for many years (e.g., Rutter, Graham, & Yule, 1970), but the reasons for the relationship remain unclear. Neurological or seizure-related variables have received the largest amount of study as potential causative factors (Hermann & Whitman, 1986), but few solid conclusions have been reached. Of the seizure-related factors that have been examined, those suggestive of a more severe seizure disorder (e.g., duration of the disorder, multiple types of seizures) have provided the strongest correlates of neuropsychological and behavioral disturbance (e.g., Dikmen, Matthews, & Harley, 1975; Lennox & Lennox, 1960; Schwartz & Dennerll, 1970; Tarter, 1972). Psychological and social explanations have received much less scientific attention, though recently more research has been conducted to explore the possible contributions of these factors (e.g., Whitman & Hermann, 1986; Hermann, Whitman & Dell, 1989).

This chapter examines the question of behavioral disturbance in children with seizures from the perspective of a biopsychosocial model of functioning. Rates of prevalence as well as a discussion of types of behavioral disturbance are examined. This is followed by a brief review of selected studies examining family issues unique to childhood epilepsy and the relationship between behavioral disturbance and marital functioning in families of children without seizures. Next, findings from a study of the appropriateness of a biopsychosocial model for understanding behavioral disturbance in a cohort of 6- to 12-year-old boys with seizures are summarized. A follow-up study of their functioning 2 to 3 years later is also presented. The chapter concludes with a discussion of the implications of these findings for further research and treatment.

Before proceeding, it should be highlighted that the term "children with seizures" is used to discuss these children. This term was chosen primarily to avoid confusion for the reader but also to avoid the use and promotion of terms considered pejorative, such as "epileptic children."

Incidence of Epilepsy in Children

Prevalence rates of epilepsy in children have ranged from 2.5 to 121/1000, with most estimates clustering around 4 to 6/1000 (Leviton & Cowan, 1982). Differences in prevalence by race, sex, age, and seizure type have been reported (Cowan, Bodensteiner, Leviton, & Boherty, 1989). According to some sources (e.g., Kurtzke & Kurland, 1984), approximately 50/100,000 individuals are newly diagnosed each year with a seizure disorder, with active seizures persisting (on average) for 13 years. Because approximately 90% of all cases experience their first seizure before they reach the age of 20 (Ziegler, 1982), it is important to recognize that epilepsy is predominantly a disorder of childhood and adolescence. Considering the relatively early age of onset, the lengthy duration of the disorder, and the emergence of the disorder during crucial stages of development, one can easily see the potential for damaging effects on a child's sense of self, the view of himself or herself relative to others, and the behavioral disturbances that might follow.

Incidence of Behavioral Disturbance

Throughout the medical literature, there indeed are reports that cite a high risk of behavioral disturbance among children with epilepsy. Studies from the 1940s through the 1960s reported highly variable rates of incidence ranging from 12% to 50%, depending primarily on where and how the sample of children was obtained (see, e.g., Bridge, 1949; Henderson, 1953). These figures are significantly higher than reports of incidence among children without medical problems, which usually has been estimated at about 2% (Miller, Hampe, Barrett, & Noble, 1971). In addition, in children without Medical problems, boys are referred to child guidance clinics three times as frequently as girls (Ross, 1980). Among children with seizures, however, girls have been found to have behavior problems equally often and similar to those noted for boys (Rutter et al., 1970). To date, no explanation has been offered for this differential rate of incidence. One possibility is that a discharging brain lesion exerts its effect equally on children, regardless of gender, although this has yet to be confirmed.

Rutter and his colleagues (Rutter et al., 1970) were the first to conduct a comprehensive and and systematic study of the relationship between seizures and behavioral disturbance. They evaluated children attending public schools between the ages of 9 and 11 years living on the Isle of Wight, England. After grouping the children into various diagnostic categories, they found that the highest prevalence of psychiatric disorder was among children with structural brain abnormalities, those who had seizures (58%) and those who did not (38%). Also, a higher prevalence of psychiatric disorder was found among the group of children with uncomplicated epilepsy (28%) compared to blind (17%), deaf (15%), and healthy control children (7%). From these findings they concluded that behavior disorder was at least four times more common in children who have seizures than in the general population. Though this research is now over 20 years old, it still provides the most representative data available on this topic.

To examine this issue further, Mellor, Lowit, and Hall (1974) identified 308 children with a seizure disorder (ages 5 to 13 years) who attended public school in Scotland and age- and gender-matched each with a child in his or her classroom. Using the same teacher questionnaire as Rutter et al. (1970), they found a 27% rate of behavior disorder in the seizure group versus 15% in the age- and gender-matched group of controls. Although the difference in incidence rates was not as large as that reported by Rutter et al., the rate of behavior disorder among children with seizures was nearly identical.

These are two of many studies that have looked at the incidence of behavior problems in children with seizures. Varying rates of behavior problems cited in other reports probably reflect differences in criteria for diagnosing psychopathology as well as the populations studied. In general, it appears that children with seizures show a higher rate of psychopathology—roughly 25% to 30%—than is seen in the general population.

Behavioral Subtypes

There is no single behavior disorder or cluster of disorders that is characteristic of children with seizures (see Bolter, 1986; Hoare, 1984a). The behaviors exhibited by children with seizures appear to cover the entire spectrum of behavior problems exhibited by children generally. The mere volume of studies cited in this chapter (and this is not an exhaustive listing) illustrates the wide range of behavioral features observed in children with seizure disorders. Boys and girls usually were not considered separately in these studies, so the percentage of boys versus girls who display these behaviors is unknown.

The behaviors reported in these studies appear to cluster under three major headings:

1. Anxious/fearful/withdrawn and dependent behavior (Breger, 1974; Bridge, 1949; Ferrari, Matthews, & Barabas, 1983; Hartlage, Green, & Offut, 1972; Hoare, 1984c; Holdsworth & Whitmore, 1974; Hughes & Jabbour, 1958; Livingston, 1977; Long & Moore, 1979; Margalit & Heiman, 1983; Matthews, Barabas, & Ferrari, 1982; Mellor et al., 1974; Ritchie, 1981; Stores, 1978; Stores & Piran, 1978).
2. Inattentive/hyperactive/restless (Breger, 1974; Grunberg & Pond, 1957; Hoare, 1984a; Holdsworth & Whitmore, 1974; Mellor et al.,

1974; Ounstead, 1955; Stores, 1978; Stores & Bennett-Levy, 1983; Stores, Hart, & Piran, 1978).
3. Aggressive/irritable/antisocial (Breger, 1974; Holdsworth & Whitmore, 1974; Mellor et al., 1974; Whitman, Hermann, Black, & Chhabria, 1982).

These categories of behavior are comparable to those categories derived from standardized questionnaires assessing children's behavior (e.g., the Child Behavior Checklist; Achenbach & Edelbrock, 1983), the items of which are intended to cover the wide range of maladaptive behaviors manifested by children across psychiatric classification schemas. Indeed, the behavior problems of children with seizures seem to form the same clusters of behavior as children without seizures.

Of the 63 children with seizures in the Rutter et al. (1970) study, 18 (28%) were diagnosed as having a psychiatric disorder. Of those 18 children, 8 (44%) were diagnosed as having "neurotic disorder," characterized by fearfulness, worry, and fussiness. Another 6 (33%) were diagnosed as "antisocial or conduct disorder," characterized by destructive, disobedient behavior, bullying other children, and lying. Three (17%) were diagnosed as exhibiting a "mixed disorder" (elements of conduct and neurotic disorders), and one (6%) received the diagnosis of "hyperkinetic syndrome." None of the children was identified as psychotic. Of the 8 children diagnosed as neurotic, 4 were boys and 4 were girls. Of the 9 children diagnosed as antisocial or mixed disorders, 5 were boys and 4 were girls. Again, the comparable frequencies of behavioral disturbance between boys and girls is striking despite the small sample size. Clearly, a more extensive study of behavioral subtypes is needed to clarify this issue.

It is noteworthy that no distinctive clusters of behavior or traits have yet been described for children with temporal lobe epilepsy, in contrast to descriptions of adults with that disorder (hypermorality, hypergraphia, social viscosity, religiosity, etc., as described by Bear & Fedio, 1977; Bear, Levin, Blumer, Chetham, & Ryder, 1982; Waxman & Geschwind, 1974). If not emergent in childhood, from where and when do these later difficulties emerge for adults? This theory has yet to be explained from a developmental perspective. Interestingly, many adult patients with temporal lobe epilepsy are reported to have experienced febrile seizures prior to the age of 2 years (Ounsted, Lindsey, & Norman, 1966). One explanation that has been offered as to the later development of these behavioral traits is that the damaged tissue continues to discharge erratically on a subclinical level, thereby exerting its influence on behavior. Yet one would assume that if scarred brain tissue later results in temporal lobe or limbic seizures, it should also manifest itself during a child's development as aberrant behavior or functioning. This has not been found consistently. Correlations have been reported between temporal lobe seizures and higher rates of behavior problems (e.g., Hoare, 1984a; Stores, 1978), and some investigators feel that these children are especially at risk for developing psychiatric disorder (Lindsay et al., 1979; Rutter et al., 1970; Stores, 1978; Taylor, 1975). Controlled analyses, however, have failed to demonstrate any significant differences between seizure type and measures of behavioral dysfunction and social competence (Whitman et al., 1982).

Possible Causes of Behavioral Disturbance

A number of factors have been suggested as responsible for, or contributing to, the development of behavioral difficulties in children with seizures. These include age of seizure onset, seizure frequency, type of seizure, duration of the disorder, etiology, degree of neuropsychological impairment, family discord, dependency, social stigma, fear of seizures, and low parental expectations. Medical factors by far have received the greatest amount of attention from researchers. In fact, these comprise approximately 79% of the nondemographic variables that were investigated empirically as potential risk factors during the period 1965–1985 (Whitman & Hermann, 1986). No single factor has been found consistently to produce behavioral disturbance in a child, although the likelihood apparently is greatest if a child has frank brain damage or seizures of known cause (see, e.g., Rutter et al., 1970; Bolter, 1986).

In general, factors indicative of a more severe seizure disorder (e.g., longer duration of the disorder, higher frequency of seizures) have been shown to be related to poorer neuropsychological functioning (Corbett & Trimble, 1983; Dikmen et al., 1975; Dodrill, 1981; Halstead, 1957; Hartlage & Green, 1972; Holdsworth & Whitmore, 1974; Klove & Matthews, 1974; Pond & Bidwell, 1960; Tarter, 1972), which, in turn, has been shown to be related to increased behavioral disturbance in some children (see, e.g., Camfield et al., 1984). A review of these factors is beyond the scope of this chapter although certainly germane to the topic. Hermann and Whitman (1984, 1986) have provided an extensive review of this area, and the reader is referred to their writings for additional information.

Family Variables and Behavioral Disturbance

The limited findings in studies examining seizure variables as causes of behavioral deviance have led investigators to examine the extent to which environmental variables may account for the increased incidence of behavior problems in these children. The probable impact of a dysfunctional family on the behavior of a child with seizures, like any other child, has long been recognized. Grunberg and Pond (1957), for example, reported that 60% of mothers of two groups of children with conduct disorders (i.e., those with seizures and those without) had a "disturbed attitude." Bagley (1971), who attempted to replicate and extend Grunberg and Pond's study, concluded that disturbed parental attitudes may, in fact, be responsible for the development of behavior problems in these children.

Unfortunately, there were numerous methodological shortcomings in studies conducted prior to 1980 that attempted to examine this issue. With few exceptions, family functioning was examined by interviewing only the mother about her impressions. In addition, many studies reported only psychiatric impressions of family dynamics (e.g., Bagley, 1971; Breger, 1974), employed idiosyncratic measures designed solely for a particular study (e.g., Bagley, 1971; Hauck, 1972), or relied on responses to one or two items from a questionnaire to divide subjects into groups (Hauck, 1972) or to draw conclusions (Breger, 1975). Further, the possibility that respondents may have answered in a socially desirable way on self-report measures (Ferrari et al., 1983; Long & Moore, 1979) was never examined, which is especially problematic in light of the stigma and prejudice that continue to affect individuals with seizures (Caveness & Gallup, 1980). Finally, although control groups have been included for comparative purposes since the 1950s (Grunberg & Pond, 1957), other methodological problems (e.g., lack of operationalization of variables of interest) have precluded drawing meaningful conclusions from these studies.

Major methodological improvements were introduced in an investigation of intrafamilial communication by Ritchie (1981). These included careful matching of control families, the employment of observational methods and independent raters, and the attainment of excellent interrater reliability. Ritchie videotaped structured family problem-solving sessions of 15 families with a child who had seizures and 15 healthy control families. In every case the child who had seizures was the oldest of the two children, was on monotherapy (Phenytoin) for seizure control, and had been seizure-free for at least 6 months. Analysis of the videotapes revealed that communication styles in families with children who had seizures were significantly different from controls. In 12 out of 15 of the patient families, the mother exerted more authority than control mothers. They also made significantly more "speeches" than their husbands, who did not differ from control fathers. The child with seizures was not as involved in the decision-making process as was the matched control; siblings in the two groups of families did not differ. Patient families, however, were generally better at solving problems than controls. They did this by "minimizing disagreements and interruptions between family members and by a greater tendency to change individual opinions in the direction of group consensus" (p. 70).

Ritchie questioned the need for such problem-solving efficiency. She noted that this interactional style was similar to that found by O'Connor (1969) in families with a mentally retarded child. According to Ritchie, O'Connor postulated that this style served to "protect the family against the potentially disruptive effect of the child's handicap" (1981, p. 70). As Ritchie noted, however, none of these children had experienced seizures for at least 6 months, and she suggested that the continued adherence to this problem-solving style ultimately could be detrimental to the child's social development. She noted that this interactive style also has been found to differentiate families of healthy children with behavior problems from those without behavior problems, and she suggested that this kind of interactive style, though adaptive for dealing with short-term crises, may create problems if maintained beyond periods of crisis. Unfortunately, Ritchie did not provide information concerning these children's behavioral functioning (i.e., assessments using standardized checklists).

In an attempt to evaluate whether epilepsy, and the family's reaction to it, is unique from other chronic disorders of childhood, Ferrari et al. (1983) evaluated 15 children with seizures, 15 with juvenile diabetes, and 15 without chronic illness, along with their parents. Compared to both control groups, children with seizures were rated by their parents as more assaultive toward them and more likely to "follow" rather than "lead," to complain about themselves, to act immaturely, and to become emotionally upset. These families described themselves as significantly less close than controls, and the content of communications "different," in that their communications frequently concerned specific issues of potential problems (e.g., someone telling secrets about the child with seizures), whereas the two control groups reported discussions of more general issues (e.g., discussion of the day's activities). The children perceived themselves to be more troublesome to their families than did controls. The children with seizures were found to have significantly lower self-concept than children with diabetes, who obtained lower scores than healthy children. From these findings, Ferrari and colleagues concluded that the presence of seizures in children "places the family at risk for problems involving family communication, cohesion, and integration" (p. 57). They concluded that these problems did not simply result from rearing a child living with a chronic illness because diabetic children and their families did not differ from healthy controls. In addition, they suggested that the lack of cohesion, communication difficulties, and poor integration may be "the tip of the iceberg" of marital discord in families dealing with epilepsy, and they suggested the need for an epidemiological study of marital discord in these families.

In a series of studies, Hoare (1984a, 1984b) examined the prevalence of psychopathology among children with chronic epilepsy and those who were newly diagnosed, comparing their rates of prevalence to children with chronic and newly diagnosed diabetes as well as to their siblings.

In all comparisons, children with seizures, whether newly diagnosed or chronic, were found to have increased rates of psychopathology compared to children with diabetes or healthy controls. In addition, siblings of the children with chronic epilepsy had higher rates of psychopathology than did siblings of the newly diagnosed group, suggesting that the mental health of siblings of children with chronic epilepsy may be adversely affected over time. An increased rate of disturbance also was found among mothers of the children with seizures. Although these studies did not address *how* these children, siblings, and mothers might become disturbed, they suggested that the disturbance seen in the behavior of the child is probably occurring in the context of disturbed familial relations.

Relationship Between Marital Discord and Behavioral Disturbance in Families of Children Without Seizures

That child behavior problems are evident when familial relations are stressed is a finding not unique to epilepsy. It is well known that behavior problems are frequently seen in children who have maritally discordant parents (Barusch & Wilcox, 1944; Emery, 1982; Porter, 1981). In fact, investigations consistently have demonstrated such a relationship using samples of children and their parents from a variety of sources. These have included children of separation and divorce (Jacobsen, 1978; Nye, 1957), children whose parents are seeking marital therapy (Porter & O'Leary, 1980), children referred to child guidance clinics (Emery & O'Leary, 1982), those who were overtly rejected from the family and placed in foster homes (Pemberton & Benady, 1973), delinquent adolescents (Duncan, 1971), and in samples unselected for either behavior problems in the child or marital discord in the parents (Block, Block, & Morrison, 1981). Some investigators have gone so far as to assert that whenever there is a problem child there is also a problem marriage (Framo, 1975).

Many theories have been advanced to explain why behavior problems in children and their parents' marital discord come to be associated. Possible mechanisms are the effects of modeling (Bandura, 1965, 1973), withdrawal of affection or extinction of social reinforcement (Patterson & Reid, 1975), inconsistent discipline or extreme parenting styles (McCord, McCord, & Howard, 1961), interparental disagreement concerning child rearing (Block et al., 1981), and others (see Emery, 1982, for a review). Disciplinary inconsistency has been demonstrated to be related to aggression and conduct problems in medically healthy boys (McCord et al., 1961). Cole and Morrow (1976) noted that marital discord between parents may preclude successful management of a behavior problem or even agreement about which behaviors are problematic. Hetherington, Stouwie, and Ridberg (1971) found that in both divorced and intact families, successful handling of the children was related to agreement between parents on disciplinary practices. Further, Block et al. (1981) found parental disagreement concerning child rearing to be related to decreased self-control in healthy boys. This relationship was demonstrated at 3, 4, and 7 years of age. In addition, they found discrepant attitudes about child rearing to be predictive of both divorce and future child behavior problems.

Marital functioning in general, and specifically agreement about parenting, has not been examined systematically in relation to the behavior displayed by children with seizures. Unfortunately, the extensive body of literature relating marital discord and child behavior problems in healthy children has not been incorporated into the research on epilepsy. To some, ameliorating parent's marital dysfunction may not seem as important a goal as seizure control when treating a child with seizures. However, these factors can be intimately intertwined; behavior problems in children with seizures have been found to be associated with disrupted marital status (divorced/separated parents) (Hermann et al., 1989) and parental disharmony has been demonstrated to have a very clear negative impact on medication compliance and therefore seizure control. Friedman et al. (1986) demonstrated that parental disharmony, based on both parental and adolescents' report, was significantly related to medication noncompliance. Obviously, the most carefully considered medication regimen will not reduce seizure frequency if other factors preclude the medication from ever becoming ingested. How a child's behavioral functioning might, in turn, be affected was not addressed in this study, but it did suggest that a multidimensional approach is needed for the successful treatment and understanding of epilepsy.

A Biopsychosocial Approach to Understanding Behavioral Disturbance in Children with Seizures

Although factors related to the seizure disorder (e.g., duration), the child's personal characteristics (e.g., neuropsychological functioning), and influences from the environment (e.g., family discord) have all been acknowledged to shape the behavior that a child with seizures ultimately displays, these factors seldom have been examined simultaneously in the same sample of children to assess their relative importance. Bruce Hermann, Steven Whitman, and colleagues have urged the consideration of a multietiological model of psychopathology and social competence in children with epilepsy and have been the primary proponents of this point of view (1986; Hermann, Whitman, Hughes, Melyn, & Dell, 1988). Their multietiological model stresses the importance of biological, psychosocial, medication, and demographic variables in accounting for the behavioral adjustment in this group of children.

In this model, high-risk variables for psychopathology include biological variables such as age at seizure onset, seizure control, duration of the disorder, seizure type, multiple seizure types, etiology, type of aura, neuropsychological status, and EEG characteristics. Psychosocial variables include parents' marital state, perceived stigma, perceived discrimination, adjustment to epilpsy, locus of control, social support, socioeconomic status, and childhood home environment. Medication variables include number of medications, serum level, medication type, and folic acid level. Demographic variables include descriptors such as age, sex, and race. This model has been supported empirically (Hermann et al., 1988). Hermann et al. found that a lack of good seizure control, a disrupted parental marriage (e.g., divorced vs. intact), male gender, younger age at onset, and the use of carbamazepine all predicted externalized behavioral disturbance (accounting for 27% of the variance), whereas internalized problems were predicted by lack of good seizure control, a disrupted parental marriage, and male gender (accounting for 23% of the variance).

The systems theory approach originally proposed by von Bertalanffy (1968) and subsequently elaborated into a biopsychosocial model by Engel (1977, 1980) also emphasizes the importance of simultaneously examining multiple spheres of functioning (biological, psychological, social) when considering a patient's psychological adjustment, response to treatment, medical status, and so on. It has achieved wide acceptance as an appropriate model for understanding many disease states (e.g., Calobrisi, 1983; Temoshock, 1985; VanderPlate, 1984; Vasile et al., 1987). This model is comparable to the systems and social-ecological model of adaptation and challenge proposed by Kazak (1989) for families of chronically ill children.

Engle's biopsychosocial model differs from Hermann and colleagues' multietiological model primarily in that the former is discussed in terms of a dynamic, ever-changing balance among the different spheres of functioning, whereas discussions of the latter do not consider this aspect (e.g., Hermann et al., 1988). It is a model specific to explaining psychopathology or social competence in epilepsy, whereas the biopsychosocial model was developed for describing behavior in medical patients generally. Nevertheless, the two models are similar in their multidimensional perspective.

In the research described in this section, the biopsychosocial model was chosen as the framework around which to examine the variables of interest primarily because of the widespread use and understanding of the model. Also, neurocognitive or intellectual status was designated as a psychological rather than a biological variable (as in Hermann et al.'s classification).

A Test of the Biopsychosocial Model

The study described here was designed to assess the appropriateness of a biopsychosocial model in accounting for the increased incidence of behavioral disturbance in boys with seizures. Additional data also were collected to assess the stability of predictor variables across time. After a review of the research literature, it was apparent that biological (seizure-related) factors, psychological (neuropsychological and/or intellectual) factors, and social (family/marital) factors had all been found to be associated with behavioral disturbance in this group of children, though rarely examined simultaneously in the same study. It was also apparent that of the three areas of functioning that comprise the biopsychosocial model, the influence of social factors had not received the same level of attention as the seizure-related factors or the contributions of the child's neuropsychological status. Of particular interest, then, was whether factors related to parenting and marital harmony were sufficiently strong to emerge as significant predictors of behavior problems in these children once the effects of neurocognitive status and seizure-related factors were controlled. Again, Hermann et al. (1988) examined the contribution of the parent's marital status in explaining the child's adjustment, but only with respect to whether the parents' were married, divorced or separated, or never married. In this study, we chose to examine parental and marital harmony at a closer level. Compared to the seizure-related variables, how important are they? To what extent is the child's neurocognitive status related to behavioral disturbance?

Sample

Because many studies have demonstrated that boys and girls react differently to marital distress, this sample consisted only of boys between the ages of 6 and 12, diagnosed as having a seizure disorder, who were otherwise healthy, had an estimated Full Scale IQ greater than or equal to 80, and were from an intact, two-parent family. These criteria were imposed so that the sample comprised as homogeneous a group of children as possible, and so that the findings would be as specific to epilepsy as possible and not attributable to other factors such as mental retardation or physical handicaps. A total of 44 children and their parents participated in the study; the data from 40 were used in the analyses. The 4 children excluded from the analyses included 2 whose parents' first language was not English and who were unable to complete the measures, 1 whose father's measures were invalid, and 1 whose diagnosis was later changed from seizures to syncopal attacks. All of the children except 1 were obtained through the neurology services at either Newington Children's Hospital (Newington, Connecticut), Yale–New Haven Hospital (New Haven, Connecticut), or University Hospital (Stony Brook, New

York). One additional child was obtained with the help of the Epilepsy Association of Long Island.

The group had a mean age of 9 years. Seven of the children had repeated a school grade; two were in special classes for gifted children. Eleven children were described by their parents as learning disabled or attending special education classes; another nine obtained remedial help in one or more subjects. Thus half of the sample was receiving some additional help in school, although the majority (73%) were attending regular classes for most of the day.

The children took a range of anticonvulsant medications, with the majority on monotherapy (n = 27, 57%). Three of the children had recently been taken off their anticonvulsant medication. In this sample of 40 children there were 20 different medication regimens.

Procedures

There were five kinds of data collected on each child and his parents: (1) parents rated their child's behavior; (2) parents rated their satisfaction in their marriage; (3) parents completed card sorts indicating attitudes and beliefs about parenting their son with seizures; (4) each child received a neuropsychological screening evaluation; and (5) relevant medical and demographic information was collected.

Behavioral functioning was obtained by having each parent complete the Child Behavior Checklist (CBCL; Achenbach & Edelbrock, 1983), a widely used measure of child psychopathology. The CBCL consists of 118 behavior problem items that are scored according to a 0 to 2 format (not true, sometimes true, often true). Factor analysis has demonstrated that this instrument consists of two broad-band scales of externalizing versus internalizing behavior problems, as well as additional narrow-band subscales. This measure has excellent psychometric properties and had been used previously in research on children with seizures (Dorenbaum, Cappelli, Keene, & McGrath, 1985; Hermann et al., 1988; Whitman et al., 1982). Each parent was asked to complete this measure without consulting his or her spouse.

Two measures of marital functioning were obtained from each parent. The first, the Locke-Wallace Marital Adjustment Test (Locke & Wallace, 1959), is a widely used 15-item self-report questionnaire that provides a global rating of marital satisfaction. It has been used by many research groups to differentiate distressed from nondistressed marital relationships (e.g., Birchler & Webb, 1977; Birchler, Weiss, & Vincent, 1975). The second measure, the Child-Rearing Practices Report (Block et al., 1981), is an objective index of parental agreement and was used to assess the extent to which parents share the same attitudes and beliefs about raising their child. It consists of a 91-item card sort which parents complete independently. The degree to which they agree in their attitudes about parenting is determined by correlating their card sorts, that is, each husband's with his wife's. This measure has excellent psychometric properties and has been found to predict divorce and child behavior problems (Block et al., 1981).

Each child's cognitive functioning was examined with a brief battery of measures assessing intellectual, perceptual, motoric, and linguistic abilities. This included an abbreviated administration of the Wechsler Intelligence Scale for Children–Revised (Vocabulary, Block Design, Picture Arrangement, and Arithmetic subtests as suggested by Kaufman, 1979), Developmental Test of Visual-Motor Integration (Beery, 1982), Grooved Pegboard (Klonoff & Low, 1974), Finger Oscillation Test (Halstead, 1947), Verbal Fluency (Gaddes & Crockett, 1975), the Jordan Left–Right Reversal Test (Jordan, 1980), and a lateral dominance exam. The children varied in their ability to execute the tasks given to them during a neuropsychological screening examination. Generally speaking, 75% of the children were able to complete the tasks within normal limits expected for their age. For the most part, children who had significant difficulty with one task experienced difficulty with the others as well. Prorated IQ scores (discussed later) ranged from 80 to 144, with a mean of 106 (SD = 17.5).

Information about the history of the child's seizure disorder (e.g., age of seizure onset, type of seizure, severity of the seizure disorder, medication, frequency of seizure activity) and descriptions of the seizure activity were obtained from the parents on an extensive questionnaire that they completed prior to their appointment. In addition, a seizure frequency and severity rating scale (Cramer et al., 1983) was used to quantify simple, complex, and secondarily generalizing partial seizures and primary generalizing tonic-clonic seizures. This measure was modified to assess absence seizures as well. The format provides both a numerical score for the frequency and severity rating of individual types of seizures and a listing of the number of seizures that occurred during the past year.

Finally, information from the child's medical record, such as electroencephalographic (EEG) findings, medication history and regimen, seizure descriptions, and seizure control on medication, was also collected. Each child's seizure disorder was then classified by an experienced epileptologist (Richard H. Mattson, M. D., West Haven VA Medical Center and Yale University) according to the Revised International Classification of Epileptic Seizures (Dreiffus et al., 1981). Approximately half of the children were classified as having primary generalizing seizures and half had partial seizures, some of whose seizures generalized.

All parents were invited to participate in the study through personal contact with their child's physician, either by telephone or by mail. The inducement for their participation in the study was that their child would receive a brief neuropsychological screening, the results of which would be discussed with them and provided to their physician, highlighting any

Table 4.1. Breakdown of children with deviant behavior ($n = 16$) (exceeding 90th percentile) as measured by the CBCL.

Internalizers	Externalizers	Mixed Disorders
3	3	10

Note. As defined by Achenbach and Edelbrock (1983), "internalizer" is used to describe a child who scores above the 98th percentile on the internalizing subscale, with that score at least 10 *t*-score points above the externalizing subscale. "Externalizer" is used to describe a child who scores above the 98th percentile on the externalizing subscale, with the score at least 10 *t*-score points above the internalizing subscale score. "Mixed disorder" is used to describe a child who scores above the 98th percentile on either the internalizing or externalizing subscale but does not have 10 *t*-score points between scores to be classified as internalizers or externalizers.

behavioral or learning difficulties observed. Contact with each family lasted between 2 and 3 hours; all data were obtained during one session.

Results

The results from the Child Behavior Checklist revealed that 16 out of the 40 boys (40%) were rated by their parents as deviant; that is, their total behavior problem scores exceeded the clinical cutoff raw score of 40 (90th percentile). No characteristic behavioral profile emerged for this group. (See Table 4.1.)

Based on previous research with adults (e.g., Batzel, Dodrill, & Fraser, 1980; Dikmen & Morgan, 1980; Dodrill, 1980; Ferguson et al., 1969) and children (Camfield et al., 1984; Hermann, 1982), it was expected that children with poorer cognitive functioning would show more behavior problems. For the purpose of these analyses, estimated Full Scale IQ was used as a global index of neurocognitive status, although its limitations are appreciated.

When IQ scores between the extreme behavioral groups were compared, significant differences were apparent. In all cases, those children who were better adjusted had higher IQs. Mean IQ score for the group with the fewest behavior problems was 109.85 ($SD = 17.16$); mean IQ score for the group with the most behavior problems was 97.61 ($SD = 14.84$; $t(38) = 2.20$; $p < .034$). A similar result was found for estimated Verbal and Performance IQ indices. The correlation between IQ and behavioral disturbance for the entire group of children was highly significant ($r = -.52$, $p < .001$).

Seizure-related variables were also found to be related to the presence of behavioral disturbance. Total seizures experienced during a child's lifetime (excluding absence seizures) was positively correlated with behavioral disturbance ($r = .44, p < .01$), as was the rating of the severity of the child's seizure disorder during the year prior to study ($r = .36, p < .05$). The number of months since the child's last seizure was negatively correlated, as expected ($r = -.34, p < .05$). Age at seizure onset was not associated with behavioral disturbance ($r = -.24, p < .05$).

To examine how child behavior problems and marital discord were related, the data were divided according to child behavior ratings falling at the two extremes on the CBCL—the top and bottom quartiles, or those who were most behaviorally disturbed and those who were not. A clear finding emerged: the deviant children had parents who disagreed more about parenting. The marital satisfaction scores also reflected greater discord among parents of children with more behavior problems, but this finding did not reach statistical significance ($p < .06$).

Multiple regression analyses were conducted in examining the relative influence of the different variables in predicting behavior problem scores. Externalized (e.g., hyperactive, aggressive, delinquent) and internalized (e.g., anxious, depressive, withdrawn) behavior problems were examined separately.

Parent's ratings of externalized behavior problems were not found to differ, so the average of their scores was used for each child. A hierarchical regression approach was used to examine whether disagreements about parenting would account for unique variance in externalized behavior problem scores once the influence of neurocognitive status and seizure-related factors was eliminated. This approach allowed for a test of the biopsychosocial model while concurrently allowing an assessment of the independent contribution of parenting disagreements. These results are presented in Table 4.2. Briefly, neurocognitive status, entered first into the multiple regression equation, accounted for 30% of the variance ($p < .0002$). The simple correlation between these two variables was $-.55$ ($p < .001$). Of the seizure-related factors, the total number of seizures the child has experienced during his lifetime correlated most highly with externalized behavior ($r = .53, p < .001$). It was entered next into the equation and accounted for an incremental 14% of the variance ($p < .004$). Disagreement about parenting accounted for an additional 13% of the variance ($p < .001$). Its correlation with externalized behavior ratings was $-.55$ ($p < .001$). Taken together, these three variables accounted for 54% of the total variance (adjusted for shrinkage).

Weaker findings emerged from analysis of internalized behavior problem scores. Data for mothers and fathers were analyzed separately because the ratings were found to differ significantly (mean score for mothers = 17.28, $SD = 10.0$; mean score for fathers = 13.0, $SD = 8.12$; $t(78) = -2.10, p < .05$). As was true for externalized scores, neurocognitive status was inversely related to mothers' ratings of internalized behavioral problems, although not as strongly ($r = -.38, p < .01$); the

Table 4.2. Hierarchical regression analysis[a] of neurocognitive, seizure-related, and parental agreement on externalized behavior problem scores.

Variable	Multiple R	R^2	R^2 IQ[b]	R^2 IQ + FREQLIFE[c]	R^2 FREQLIFE	R^2 IQ + FREQLIFE + QSORT[d]	R^2 QSORT	F change	Significance of R^2
Estimated Full Scale IQ scores	.55	.30 (.28)	.30 (.28)					16.39	$p < .0002$
Total seizures experienced in lifetime	.67			.44 (.41)	.14 (.13)			9.38	$p < .004$
Q-sort scores	.76					.58 (.54)	.13 (.13)	11.28	$p < .001$

[a] Adjusted R^2 scores following allowance for shrinkage are presented in parentheses underneath unadjusted R^2 scores.
[b] IQ = estimated Full Scale IQ.
[c] FREQLIFE = number of seizures experienced during the child's lifetime.
[d] QSORT = degree of correlation between parents on card-sorting task.

same correlation using fathers' ratings failed to reach significance. Seizure severity during the year prior to study was significantly related to mothers' ratings ($r = .36$, $p < .05$), but not fathers'. Disagreement about parenting was not related to mothers' or fathers' ratings of internalized behaviors. When entered into regression analyses using mothers' ratings, neurocognitive status accounted for 14% of the variance in behavior problem scores ($p < .02$). Severity of the seizure disorder during the year prior to study accounted for an incremental 8.8% of the variance ($p < .05$). Regression analyses were not performed using fathers' ratings of internalized behavior given that these did not correlate significantly with any of the variables of interest.

Discussion

Disagreements about parenting a boy with seizures were found to be related to externalized behavior problems in these boys, accounting for about as much of the variance as seizure-related variables. Self-reports of global marital discord were not related to the report of behavior problems, although the trend in the data suggested that with a larger sample this may have been found. More generally, all spheres tested within the model (e.g., the biological, psychological, and social) were related to the presence of behavior problems, with overall neurocognitive status (as reflected by IQ) accounting for the largest proportion of the variance. Thus the appropriateness of this model for accounting for externalized behavior problems in children with seizures was supported.

Given the volume of research that has been generated in search of the medical variables that are most responsible for the increased behavioral deviance in children with seizures, it is especially noteworthy that disagreement about parenting accounted for about as much of the variance in externalized behavior problem scores as the seizure-related variables. This point by itself warrants highlighting, because medical factors are typically thought of as causative when a child with seizures also has behavioral difficulties. It suggests psychosocial intervention may be at least as appropriate as medical intervention for some children.

The relationship between behavioral disturbance and parenting disagreement may be true only for externalized behaviors (e.g., hyperactivity, aggression, delinquency) and not internalized ones (e.g, depression, anxiety, withdrawal). This finding would call into question any reports that failed to make this distinction, instead reporting total or summary scores of behavioral disturbance or psychopathology. Moreover, fathers may not be as reliable as mothers in reporting behavior problems unless an externalized or disruptive behavior problem is present.

This study represented the first attempt to use parental disagreement as a predictor of behavioral outcome in children with seizures. Hermann et al. (1988) also found that parents' marital status predicted child behavioral outcome. Taken together, these findings suggested that multiple realms of functioning, including marriage-related issues, must be considered when the etiology of child behavior problems is examined.

A notable omission in the research on behavioral disturbance in children with seizures is the lack of longitudinal data. As of this writing, there are no studies that have examined across an extended time period the course of behavior disorders in this group of children (with the exception of the study presented next). Is there predictive utility in knowing that a child's parents disagree about parenting? Does neurocognitive status predict how a child will behave several years later? If a child has had an excessive number of seizures, does this mean that he is likely to have persistent behavioral difficulties? The following study attempted to answer these questions.

Follow-Up Study

To assess the stability of the findings over time and to assess whether future behavior could be predicted by any of the factors identified in the initial study, families were recontacted $2\frac{1}{2}$ to 3 years later and invited to participate in a mail and telephone follow-up concerning the behavioral adjustment of their sons with seizures. To my knowledge, this was the first longitudinal assessment of behavior disorders in children with seizures. Seventy-five percent of the original sample participated ($N = 30$) and completed a structured telephone questionnaire, seizure disorder severity rating scale (Cramer et al., 1983), and the CBCL. For purposes of consistency among respondents, only mothers were asked to provide all information. Chi-square analyses revealed no differential attrition of respondents on demographic or behavioral variables.

The boys ranged from 8 years, 2 months to 16 years in age at follow-up ($M = 11$ years, 6 months; $SD = 2$ years, 4 months). All attended regular schools and 47% ($n = 14$) were receiving at least some special education services. As a group, the children's estimated Full Scale IQ (based on the previously obtained assessment) was in the average range ($M = 106.4$, $SD = 18.0$). Forty percent ($n = 12$) of mothers reported that their son was no longer taking antiseizure medication, whereas this was true for only 10% ($n = 3$) of the sample initially. Sixty-three percent ($n = 19$) reported no additional seizure activity since the initial study (Time 1); 11 boys (33%) continued to have seizures since participating in the initial study, with 8 of those 11 (27%) experiencing seizures during the year prior to the follow-up study.

The number and severity of behavior problems exhibited by these boys tended to persist over the $2\frac{1}{2}$ to 3 year span (total behavior problem scores, $r = .61$, $p < .001$). Of the 30 children in the follow-up sample, 4 mothers reported behavior worsening, 9 reported improvement, and 17 reported essentially no change (as defined by at least 10 *T*-score difference between initial study and follow-up total scores on the CBCL). Seven of the boys (23%) scored in the clinically deviant range at follow-up (Time 2) as compared to 11 (36%) of these same boys during the initial study (Time 1). Of these 7 behavior disordered boys, had experienced at least one seizure since Time 1, and 6 continued to take antiseizure medication. For the entire group, 53% of mothers acknowledged at least considering the need for professional assistance to help them manage their son's behavior at home or at school, whereas 23% actually sought help.

Of the measures obtained at Time 1, only the severity of the child's seizure disorder during the year prior to study predicted Time 2 internalizing behavior problems [accounting for 22.5% of the variance; $F(1,26) = 8.85$, $p < .01$]; none of the variables of interest predicted Time 2 externalized behavior problems. Neurocognitive status and parental disagreement at Time 1, although significant Time 1 determinants of behavioral adjustment, did not predict Time 2 behavioral adjustment.

Just as factors related to the severity of seizure disorder and parental relationship factors predicted behavior problems in the initial study, these variables assessed at follow-up predicted behavioral outcome at follow-up (after the influence of previous behavior problems was apportioned). Severity of the seizure disorder was most important in predicting overall behavioral outcome, accounting for the largest proportion of the variance in total behavior problems (a combined measure of externalized and internalized problems) at Time 2 (16.5%, $p < .003$), followed by mothers' ratings of marital satisfaction (7.8%, $p < .02$). In telephone interviews, mothers' reports of parental disagreement concerning various child-rearing topics were found to be related to the number of seizures that the child experienced since Time 1 ($r = .34$, $p < .03$) and the severity of the child's seizure disorder over the past year ($r = .37$, $p < .02$). Disagreement between parents about child-rearing issues was significantly related to behavioral disturbance ($r = .45$, $p < .006$). Parental disagreement at follow-up was also significantly related to the number of major life stressors (relocation, change in financial status, death or prolonged illness of a family member, etc.) experienced by the family over the prior 2 to 3 years ($r = .30$, $p < .05$).

Overall, the boy's behavior improved from Time 1 to Time 2, as did the frequency of their seizure disorders. Thirty-six percent of these boys scored in the clinically deviant range at Time 1, whereas only 23% did at follow-up. Similarly, 37% of this sample had experienced seizures the year prior to study at Time 1, whereas this was true for 27% at Time 2.

Clearly, the most robust predictor of behavioral disturbance/adjustment, as seen through the mothers' eyes, was prior behavioral disturbance/adjustment. Whether this reflects consistency in the behavior of the children of consistency in the perspective of mothers of their children is impossible to determine without independent assessments of the children's behavior.

Discussion

Severity of the seizure disorder during the year prior to study proved to be an effective predictor of behavior, both concurrently and longitudinally. These data suggest that those children with the most persistent seizure disorders have the most persistent behavioral disturbance. This finding is consistent with those studies reported earlier that found that problems with behavior and neuropsychological functioning are associated with more severe seizure disorders.

Disagreement about parenting assessed at Time 1 failed to predict behavioral disturbance at Time 2. It appeared that parental relationship factors and family stressors were more likely a function of immediate concerns within the family, so that they predicted *concurrent* behavior problems but did not provide a stable basis for prediction over a longer time interval. This differed from findings reported by Block et al. (1981), where disagreements about parenting predicted future behavior problems in a sample of preschool children without medical concerns. Perhaps the presence of a seizure disorder in a child overpowers family relationship factors that would ordinarily predict behavioral outcome. Alternatively, perhaps with time parents feel better able to cope with their child's seizure disorder, resulting in more consistent parenting and therefore less disagreement.

It is noteworthy that the severity of the child's seizure disorder at Time 1 predicted internalized behavior problems but not externalized behavior problems. One possible explanation for this finding is that as the child matured, he became more worried about the possibility of having seizures and became fearful/anxious as a result of experiencing the negative reactions of others to seizures. Certainly, low self-esteem and fear of seizures have been described as prominent in individuals with seizures (e.g., Ferrari et al., 1983; Mittan, 1986). This scenario suggests that the biological and social factors may converge to create psychological disturbance in the child, though a change in any one sphere of functioning could result in concomitant changes in the others.

Implications for Further Research and Treatment

More research is needed to elucidate the associations involving family functioning, neuropsychological functioning of the child with seizures, factors related to the severity of the seizure disorder, and the child's behavioral functioning. Longitudinal studies that identify children at the time of diagnosis with future follow-up not only of the child's functioning but of the family's functioning as well would contribute significantly to our understanding of the interrelationship among these variables. The effects of anticonvulsants on behavior and cognition might also be much better understood within such a framework.

The findings presented in this chapter must be applied cautiously to groups that deviate from the study's selection criteria. It must be remembered that these were all elementary school–aged boys with seizures who were generally within the normal range of intellectual functioning, without other medical illness or physical handicap, and were from intact, two-parent families. It is not clear how the findings may differ for girls, adolescents, handicapped youngsters, or children from single-parent families. Further refinements might include, obtaining observational data about the parents' communication abilities and marital discord, identifying the precise areas where disagreements about parenting arise, and securing multiple raters (e.g., teachers) of the child's behavior.

The findings from these studies raise some important issues concerning treatment of the child with seizures. They suggest that medically treating the child's seizure disorder when the child's behavior is also a problem is not the only option for the pediatrician or pediatric neurologist. A referral for therapy (e.g., family, marital, individual) may not only be helpful; it may be a critical avenue for intervention. Similarly, mental health professionals treating children with seizures and behavior problems need to consider possible influences on behavior of the child's neurological disorder as well as disagreements about parenting. Family education about epilepsy or family therapy may be indicated. For example, helping parents understand what seizures are and what they are not, dispelling myths about epilepsy, helping them learn how to answer family's and friends' questions about their child with seizures, and generally helping parents to cope with their child's disorder may reduce disagreements about how to effectively parent, which, in turn, may reduce behavioral disturbance in the child.

Tavriger (1966) found that approximately one-third of parents of children with seizures rejected scientific explanations about the etiology and exacerbation of seizure disorders and instead endorsed their own ideas of how seizures emerged. In an apparent attempt to control the seizures, the majority of parents blamed their child's seizure disorder on prolonged stress (such as anxiety over quarrelling parents or relatives), depression/unhappiness over separation, bad parental relationships, or feeling upset. Thus educating parents about those aspects of epilepsy that they can control and those they cannot may help toward establishing more consistent parenting practices.

Helping the family and the patient to develop healthy intrafamilial communication through family therapy may decrease the likelihood of the child developing low self-esteem and fearful or anxious behavior secondary to the seizure disorder. Ziegler (1981) presented a model of family functioning that describes how parents can easily become over-protective as they attempt to allay feelings of guilt or responsibility for the seizures. He also offers an approach to psychotherapeutic intervention that incorporates this model into therapeutic practice and highlights different modes of intervention appropriate to these families, depending on the particular circumstances involved (Ziegler, 1982).

Though the incidence of behavioral disturbance is elevated in this group relative to the general population of children, the causes are clearly multiple and not solely medical. For neuropsychologists and others involved with the assessment and treatment of children with seizures, the present findings should underscore the importance of psychosocial factors. Also, the findings from the longitudinal study highlight the need for ongoing assessment (and intervention) of children with seizures and their parents, in that the influence of parenting decisions on a child's behavior may not be a stable predictor of behavioral adjustment across a 2 to 3 year time period. Clearly, controlled research is needed to validate these assertions and to replicate the current findings.

The various associations found in this body of research literature involving neuropsychological, behavioral, environmental, and medical factors highlight the inadequacies of reductionistic models in accounting for difficulties encountered by children with seizures and their families. In research and in treatment, a multietiologic (Hermann & Whitman, 1986) or biopsychosocial model (Engel, 1977, 1980) must be considered, along with the recognition that factors influencing a child's behavior are not static and are likely to change over time.

Acknowledgment. The author gratefully acknowledges the expertise offered and contributions made to this research by R. C. Delaney, Ph.D., and R. H. Mattson, M.D., West Haven VA Medical Center and Yale University; G. Holmes, M.D., Boston Children's Hospital and Harvard University; M. G. Tramontana, Ph.D., Vanderbilt University; and K. D. O'Leary, Ph.D., State University of New York at Stony Brook.

References

Achenbach, T. M., & Edelbrock, C. S. (1983). *Manual for the The Child Behavior Checklist and Revised Child Behavior Profile*. Burlington, VT: Queen City Printers.

Bagley, C. (1971). *The social psychology of the child with epilepsy*. London: Routledge & Kegan Paul.

Bandura, A. (1965). *Principles of behavior modification* New York: Holt, Rinehart & Winston.

Bandura, A. (1973). *Aggression: A social learning approach*. Englewood Cliffs, NJ: Prentice-Hall.

Barusch, D. W., & Wilcox, J. A. (1944). A study of sex differences in preschool children's adjustment coexistent with interparental tensions. *Journal of Genetic Psychology*, *64*, 281–303.

Batzel, L. W., Dodrill, C. B., & Fraser, R. T. (1980). Further validation of the WSPI Vocational Scale: Comparisons with other correlates of employment in epilepsy. *Epilepsia*, *21*, 235–242.

Bear, D. M., & Fedio, P. (1977). Quantitative analysis of interictal behavior in temporal lobe epilepsy. *Archives of Neurology*, *34*, 454–467.

Bear, D. M., Levin, K., Blumer, D., Chetham, D., & Ryder, J. (1982). Interictal behavior in hospitalized temporal lobe epileptics: Relationship to idiopathic psychiatric syndromes. *Journal of Neurology, Neurosurgery and Psychiatry*, *45*, 481–485.

Beery, K. (1982). *Manual for the Developmental Test of Visual-Motor Integration*. Cleveland, OH: Modern Curriculum Press.

Birchler, G. R., & Webb, L. J. (1977). Discriminating interaction behaviors in happy and unhappy marriages. *Journal of Consulting and Clinical Psychology*, *45*, 494–495.

Birchler, G. R., Weiss, R. L., & Vincent, J. P. (1975). Multimethod analysis of social reinforcement exchange between maritally distressed and non-distressed spouse and stranger dyads. *Journal of Personality and Social Psychology*, *31*, 349–360.

Block, J. H., Block, J., & Morrison, A. (1981). Parental agreement–disagreement on child-rearing orientations and gender-related personality correlates in children. *Child Development*, *52*, 965–974.

Bolter, J. F. (1986). Epilepsy in children: Neuropsychological effects. In J. E. Obrzut & G. W. Hynd (Eds.), *Child neuropsychology: Vol. 2. Clinical practice* (pp. 59–81). Orlando, FL: Academic Press.

Bourgeois, B. F. D., Prensky, A. L., Palkes, H. S., Talent, B. K., & Busch, S. G. (1983). Intelligence in epilepsy: A prospective study in children. *Annals of Neurology*, *14*, 438–444.

Breger, E. (1974). Psychiatric consultation to the epileptic child and his family: A study of 60 cases. Part 2. *Maryland State Medical Journal*, *26*, 39–44.

Breger, E. (1975). Parental over-protection and rejection: Implications for the epileptic child. *Maryland State Medical Journal*, *26*, 63–67.

Bridge, E. M. (1949). *Epilepsy and convulsive disorders in children*. New York: McGraw-Hill.

Calobrisi, A. (1983). Biopsychosocial study of diabetes mellitus. *Psychotherapy and Psychosomatics*, *39*, 193–200.

Camfield, P. R., Gates, R., Ronen, G., Camfield, C., Ferguson, M. A., & MacDonald, G. W. (1984). Comparison of cognitive ability, personality profile, and school success in epileptic children with pure right versus left temporal lobe EEG foci. *Annals of Neurology*, *15*, 122–126.

Caveness, W. F., & Gallup, G. H. (1980). A survey of public attitudes toward epilepsy in 1979 with an indication of trends over the past thirty years. *Epilepsia*, *21*, 509–518.

Cole, C., & Morrow, W. R. (1976). Refractory parent behaviors in behavior modification training groups. *Psychotherapy, Research & Practice*, *13*, 162–169.

Corbett, J. A., & Trimble, M. R. (1983). Epilepsy and anticonvulsant medication. In M. Rutter (Ed.), *Developmental neuropsychiatry* (pp. 112–129). London: Guilford Press.

Cowan, L. D., Bodensteiner, J. B., Leviton, A., & Doherty, L. (1989). Prevalence of the epilepsies in children and adolescents. *Epilepsia*, *30*, 94–106.

Cramer, J. A., Smith, D. B., Mattson, R. H., Escueta, A. V. D., Collins, J. F., and the VA Cooperative Study Group (1983). A method of quantification for the evaluation of anti-epileptic drug therapy. *Neurology*, *33*(Suppl. 1), 26–37.

Dikmen, S., Matthews, C. G., & Harley, J. P. (1975). The effect of early versus late onset of major motor epilepsy upon cognitive-intellectual performance. *Epilepsia*, *16*, 73–81.

Dikmen, S., & Morgan, S. F. (1980). Neuropsychological factors related to employability and occupational status in persons with epilepsy. *Journal of Nervous and Mental Diseases*, *168*, 236–240.

Dodrill, C. B. (1980). Interrelationships between neuropsychological data and social problems in epilepsy. In R. Canger, F. Angeleri, & J. K. Penry (Eds.), *Advances in epileptology: XIth Epilepsy International Symposium* (pp. 191–197). New York: Raven Press.

Dodrill, C. B. (1981). Neuropsychology of epilepsy. In S. B. Filskov & T. J. Boll (Eds.), *Handbook of clinical neuropsychology* (pp. 366–395). New York: Wiley.

Dodrill, C. B. (1986). Correlates of generalized tonic-clonic seizures with intellectual, neuropsychological, emotional, and social function in patients with epilepsy. *Epilepsia*, *27*, 399–411.

Dorenbaum, D., Cappelli, H. B. A., Keene, D., & McGrath, P. J. (1985). Use of a Child Behavior Checklist in the psychosocial assessment of children with epilepsy. *Clinical Pediatrics*, *24*, 634–637.

Dreifuss, F. E., Penry, J. K., Bancaud, J., Henricksen, O., Rubio-Donadieu, F., & Steins, M. (1981). Proposal for revised clinical and electroencephalographic classification of epileptic seizures. *Epilepsia*, *22*, 489–501.

Duncan, O. D. (1971). Parental attitudes and interactions in delinquency. *Child Development*, *42*, 1751–1765.

Emery, R. E. (1982). Interparental conflict and the children of discord and divorce. *Psychological Bulletin*, *92*, 310–330.

Emery, R. E., & O'Leary, K. D. (1982). Children's perceptions of marital discord and behavior problems of boys and girls. *Journal of Abnormal Child Psychology*, *10*, 11–24.

Engel, G. L. (1977). The need for a new medical model: A challenge for biomedicine. *Science*, *196*, 129–136.

Engel, G. L. (1980). The clinical application of the biopsychosocial model. *American Journal of Psychiatry*, *137*, 535–544.

Farwell, J. R., Dodrill, C. B., & Batzell, L. W. (1985). Neuropsychological abilities of children with epilepsy. *Epilepsia*, *26*, 395–400.

Ferguson, S. M., Rayport, M., Gardner, R., Kass, W., Weiner, H., & Reiser, M. F. (1969). Similarities in mental content of psychotic states, spontaneous seizures, dreams, and responses to electrical brain stimulation in patients with temporal lobe epilepsy. *Psychosomatic Medicine*, *31*, 479–497.

Ferrari, M., Matthews, W., & Barabas, G. (1983). The family and the child with epilepsy. *Family Process*, *22*, 53–59.

Framo, J. L. (1975). Personal reflections of a therapist. *Journal of Marriage and Family Counseling*, *1*, 15–28.

Friedman, I. M., Litt, I. F., King, D. R., Henson, R., Holtzman, D., Halverson, D., & Kraemer, H. C. (1986). Compliance with anticonvulsant therapy by epileptic youth: Relationships to psychosocial aspects of adolescent development. *Journal of Adolescent Health Care*, *7*, 12–17.

Gaddes, W. H., & Crockett, D. (1975). The Spreen Benton Aphasia Tests: Normative data as a measure of normal language development. *Brain and Language*, *2*, 257–280.

Grunberg, F., & Pond, D. A. (1957). Conduct disorders in epileptic children. *Journal of Neurology, Neurosurgery and Psychiatry*, *20*, 65–68.

Halstead, H. (1957). Abilities and behavior of epileptic children. *Journal of Mental Science*, *103*, 28–47.

Halstead, W. C. (1947). *Brain and intelligence*. Chicago: University of Chicago Press.

Hartlage, L. C., & Green, J. B. (1972). The relation of parental attitudes to academic and social achievement in epileptic children. *Epilepsia*, *13*, 21–26.

Hartlage, L. C., Green, J. B., & Offutt, L. (1972). Dependency in epileptic children. *Epilepsia*, *13*, 27–30.

Hauck, G. (1972). Sociological aspects of epilepsy research. *Epilepsia*, *13*, 79–85.

Henderson, P. (1953). Epilepsy in school children. *British Journal of Preventive and Social Medicine*, *7*, 9–13.

Hermann, B. P. (1982). Neuropsychological functioning and psychopathology in children with epilepsy. *Epilepsia*, *23*, 703–710.

Hermann, B. P., & Whitman, S. (1984). Behavioral and personality correlates of epilepsy: A review, methodological critique, and conceptual model. *Psychological Bulletin*, *95*, 451–497.

Hermann, B. P., & Whitman, S. (1986). Psychopathology in epilepsy: A multietiologic model. In S. Whitman & B. P. Hermann (Eds.), *Psychopathology in epilepsy: Social dimensions* (pp. 5–37). New York: Oxford University Press.

Hermann, B. P., Whitman, S., Hughes, J. R., Melyn, M. M., & Dell, J. (1988). Multietiological determinants of psychopathology and social competence in children with epilepsy. *Epilepsy Research*, *2*, 51–60.

Hermann, B. P., Whitman, S., & Dell, J. (1989). Correlates of behavior problems and social competence in children with epilepsy, aged 6–11. In B. Hermann & M. Seidenberg (Eds.), *Childhood epilepsies: Neuropsychological, Psychosocial and Intervention aspects* (pp. 143–157). New York: John Wiley & Sons.

Hetherington, E. G., Stouwie, R. J., & Ridberg, E. H. (1971). Patterns of family interaction and child-rearing attitudes related to three dimensions of juvenile delinquency. *Journal of Abnormal Psychology*, *78*, 160–176.

Hoare, P. (1984a). The development of psychiatric disorder in schoolchildren with epilepsy. *Developmental Medicine and Child Neurology*, *26*, 3–13.

Hoare, P. (1984b). Psychiatric disturbance in the families of epileptic children. *Developmental Medicine and Child Neurology*, *26*, 14–19.

Hoare, P. (1984c). Does illness foster dependency? A study of epileptic and diabetic children. *Developmental Medicine and Child Neurology*, *26*, 20–24.

Holdsworth, L., & Whitmore, K. (1974). A study of children with epilepsy attending ordinary schools: I. Their seizure patterns, progress, and behavior in school. *Developmental Medicine and Child Neurology*, *16*, 746–758.

Hughes, J. G., & Jabbour, J. T. (1958). The treatment of the epileptic child. *Journal of Pediatrics*, *53*, 66–68.

Jacobson, D. S. (1978). The impact of marital separation/divorce on children: II. Interparental hostility and child adjustment. *Journal of Divorce*, *2*, 3–20.

Jordan, K. (1980). *The Jordan Left–Right Reversal Test*. Novato, CA: Academic Therapy Publications.

Kaufman, A. S. (1979). *Intelligent testing with the WISC-R*. New York: Wiley.

Kazak, A. E. (1989). Families of chronically ill children: A systems and social-ecological model of adaptation and challenge. *Journal of Consulting and Clinical Psychology*, *57*, 25–30.

Klonoff, H., & Low, M. (1974). Disordered brain function in young children and early adolescents: Neuropsychological and electroencephalographic correlates. In R. M. Reitan & L. A. Davison (Eds.), *Clinical neuropsychology* (pp. 121–178). New York: Wiley.

Klove, H., & Matthews, C. G. (1974). Neuropsychological studies of patients with epilepsy. In R. M. Reitan & L. A. Davison (Eds.), *Clinical Neuropsychology: Current Status and Applications*, Winston and Sons, Washington, DC, pp. 237–265.

Knights, R. M., & Moule, A. D. (1968). Normative data on the motor steadiness battery for children. *Perceptual and Motor Skills*, *26*, 643–650.

Kurtzke, J. F., & Kurland, L. T. (1984). The epidemiology of neurologic disease. In A. B. Baker & L. H. Baker (Eds.), *Clinical neurology* (Vol. 4, pp. 1–143). Philadelphia: Harper & Row.

Lennox, W., & Lennox, M. (1960). *Epilepsy and related disorders*. Boston: Little, Brown.

Leviton, A., & Cowan, L. D. (1982). Epidemiology of seizure disorders in children. *Neuroepidemiology*, *1*, 40–83.

Lindsay, J., Ounsted, C., & Richards, P. (1979). Long-term outcome in children with temporal lobe seizures. III. Psychiatric aspects in childhood and adult life. *Developmental Medicine and Child Neurology*, *21*, 630–636.

Livingston, S. (1977, Winter). Psychosocial aspects of epilepsy. *Journal of Clinical Child Psychology*, pp. 6–12.

Locke, H. J., & Wallace, K. M. (1959). Short marital adjustment and prediction tests: Their reliability and validity. *Marriage and the Family*, *21*, 251–255.

Long, C. G., & Moore, J. R. (1979). Parental expectations for their epileptic children. *Journal of Child Psychology and Psychiatry*, *24*, 299–312.

Margalit, M., & Heiman, T. (1983). Anxiety and self-dissatisfaction in epileptic children. *International Journal of Social Psychiatry*, *29*, 220–224.

Matthews, W. S., Barabas, G., & Ferrari, M. (1982). Emotional concomitants of childhood epilepsy. *Epilepsia*, *23*, 671–681.

McCord, W., McCord, J., & Howard, A. (1961). Familial correlates of aggression in nondelinquent male children. *Journal of Abnormal and Social Psychology*, *62*, 79–93.

Mellor, D. H., Lowit, I., & Hall, D. J. (1974). Are epileptic children behaviorally different from other children? In P. Harris & C. Mawdsley (Eds.), *Epilepsy proceedings of the Hans Breger centenary symposium* (pp. 313–316). Edinburgh: Churchill-Livingstone.

Miller, L. C., Hampe, E., Barrett, C. L., & Noble, H. (1971). Children's deviant behavior within the general population. *Journal of Consulting and Clinical Psychology*, *37*, 16–22.

Mittan, R. J. (1986). Fear of seizures. In S. Whitman & B. P. Hermann (Eds.), *Psychopathology in epilepsy: Social dimensions* (pp. 90–121). New York: Oxford University Press.

Nye, F. I. (1957). Child adjustment in broken and in unhappy, broken homes. *Marriage and Family Living*, *19*, 356–361.

O'Connor, W. A. (1969). *Patterns of interaction in families with high-adjusted, low adjusted, and retarded members*. Unpublished dissertation, University of Kansas, Lawrence.

Ounstead, C. (1955). The hyperkinetic syndrome in epileptic children. *Lancet*, *2*, 303–311.

Ounstead, C., Lindsay, J. T., & Norman, R. M. (1966). Biological factors in temporal lobe epilepsy. *Clinics in Developmental Medicine* (Vol. 22). London: Heinemann Medical Books.

Patterson, G. R., & Reid, J. B. (1975). *A social learning approach to family intervention*. Eugene, OR: Castalia Publishing Co.

Pedhazer, E. (1982). *Multiple regression in behavioral research: Explanation and prediction* (2nd ed.). New York: CBS College Publishing.

Pemberton, D. A., & Benady, D. R. (1973). Consciously rejected children. *British Journal of Psychiatry*, *123*, 575–578.

Pond, D. A., & Bidwell, B. H. (1960). A survey of epilepsy in fourteen general practices: II. Social and psychological aspects. *Epilepsia*, *1*, 285–299.

Porter, B. (1981) *Parental behavior and feelings in distressed and nondistressed marriages*. Unpublished dissertation, State University of New York at Stony Brook.

Porter, B., & O'Leary, K. D. (1980). Marital discord and childhood behavior problems. *Journal of Abnormal Child Psychology*, *80*, 287–295.

Ritchie, K. (1981). Research note: Interaction in the families of epileptic children. *Journal of Child Psychology and Psychiatry*, *22*, 65–71.

Ross, A. O. (1980). *Psychological disorders of children: A behavioral approach to theory, research and therapy*. New York: McGraw-Hill.

Rutter, M., Graham, P., & Yule, W. (1970). *A neuropsychiatric study in childhood*. Philadelphia: Lippincott.

Schwartz, M., & Dennerll, R. D. (1970). Neuropsychological assessment of children with, without, and with questionable epileptogenic dysfunction. *Perceptual and Motor Skills*, *30*, 111–121.

Stores, G. (1978). School-children with epilepsy at risk for learning and behavior problems. *Developmental Medicine and Child Nuerology*, *20*, 502–508.

Stores, G. (1981). Problems of learning and behavior in children with epilepsy. In E. H. Reynolds & M. R. Trimble (Eds.), *Epilepsy and psychiatry* (pp. 33–48). Edinburgh: Churchill-Livingstone.

Stores, G., & Bennett-Levy, J. (1983). The nature of learning difficulties in schoolchildren with epilepsy. *British Journal of Clinical Practice* (Symposium Suppl. 27), pp. 92–98.

Stores, G., Hart, J., & Piran, N. (1978). Inattentiveness in schoolchildren with epilepsy. *Epilepsia*, *19*, 169–175.

Stores, G., & Piran, N. (1978). Dependency of different types in school children with epilepsy. *Psychological Medicine*, *8*, 441–445.

Tarter, R. E. (1972). Intellectual and adaptive functioning in epilepsy: A review of fifty years of research. *Diseases of the Nervous System*, *33*, 763–770.

Taylor, D. C. (1975). Factors influencing the occurrence of schizophrenia-like Psychosis in patients with temporal lobe epilepsy. *Psychological Medicine*, *5*, 249–254.

Tavriger, R. (1986). Some parental theories about the causes of epilepsy. *Epilepsia*, *7*, 339–343.

Temoshok, L. (1985). Biopsychosocial studies on cutaneous malignant melanoma: Psychosocial factors associated with prognostic indicators, progression, psychophysiology and trmor-host response. *Social Science Medicine*, *20*, 833–840.

Tizard, B. (1962). The personality of epileptics: A discussion of the evidence. *Psychological Bulletin*, *59*, 196–210.

Trimble, M. R., & Cull, C. (1988). Children of school-age: The influence of anti-epileptic drugs on behavior and intellect. *Epilepsia*, *29*(Suppl. 3), S15–S19.

VanderPlate, C. (1984). Psychological aspects of multiple sclerosis and its treatment: Toward a biopsychosocial perspective. *Health Psychology*, *3*, 253–272.

Vasile, R. G., Samson, J. A., Bemporad, J., Bloomingdale, K. L., Creasy, D., Fenton, B. T., Gudeman, J. E., & Schildkraut, J. J. (1987). A biopsychosocial approach to treating patients with affective disorders. *American Journal of Psychiatry*, *144*, 341–344.

von Bertalanffy, L. (1968). *General systems theory*. New York: Braziller.

Waltzer, H. (1982). The biopsychosocial model for brief inpatient treatment of the schizophrenic syndrome. *Psychiatric Quarterly*, *54*, 97–108.

Waxman, S. G., & Geschwind, N. (1974). Hypergraphia in temporal lobe epilepsy. *Neurology*, *24*, 629–636.

Whitman, S., & Hermann, B. P. (Eds.) (1986). *Psychopathology in epilepsy: Social dimensions*. New York: Oxford University Press.

Whitman, S., Hermann, B. P., Blcak, R. B., & Chhabria, S. (1982). Psychopathology and seizure type in children with epilepsy. *Psychological Medicine*, *12*, 843–853.

Ziegler, R. G. (1981). Impairments of control and competence in epileptic children and their families. *Epilepsia*, *22*, 339–346.

Ziegler, R. G. (1982). The child with epilepsy: Psychotherapy and counseling. In H. Sands (Ed.), *Epilepsy: A handbook for the mental health professional* (pp. 158–188). New York: Brunner/Mazel.

CHAPTER 5

Considerations in the Use of Dichotic Listening with Children

KENNETH HUGDAHL

This chapter is concerned with the use of dichotic listening (DL) to assess language laterality and brain–behavior relationships in children. When DL has been used with children there are two main avenues of investigation (Hiscock & Decter, 1988). The first is the developmental, or ontogenetic, aspect of the phenomenon under study. In the DL case this traditionally has been focused on whether laterality develops over time (e.g., Lenneberg, 1967). The other main route is to use children to elucidate basic theoretical questions and to examine mediating mechanisms in laterality (e.g., see Kinsbourne & Hiscock, 1977).

Dichotic listening is a technique used to reveal information processing differences between the cerebral hemispheres (Hellige, 1990). In this sense, the study of DL means studying the functional specificity of cerebral organization. Dichotic performance reflects the brain's limited capacity to handle "two things at the same time," as when two messages are in cognitive conflict. Thus although DL has been used mainly to assess language laterality, in a more general sense the technique taps broad cognitive functions, like attention, perception, and memory. The use of DL in developmental studies is therefore not restricted to assessment of language function.

In this chapter, I discuss several of the uses of DL in studies of children. I also discuss the use of DL in clinical situations (e.g., when assessing cerebral dominance patterns in children with brain lesions, or before neurosurgery). In addition, I address methodological problems and shortcomings with the DL technique (see also Hugdahl, 1988). Finally, I review some data from the Somatic Psychology Laboratory at the University of Bergen, Norway, including the use of DL in investigations of cognitive function and language laterality in children (Andersson & Hugdahl, 1987; Bø, Hugdahl, & Marklund, 1989; Hugdahl & L. Andersson, 1986; Hugdahl, L. Andersson, Asbjørnsen, & Dalen, 1990), recent studies related to dyslexia and reading disorders (Hugdahl, Ellertsen, Waaler, & Kløve, 1989; Hugdahl, Synnevaag, & Satz, 1990), and studies using DL with neurological patient groups (Hugdahl, Wester, & Asbjørnsen, 1990a,b).

Developmental Shifts in Ear Advantage

The use of dichotic listening in children has been related closely to the issue of developmental changes in laterality and language functions. Because language and reading skills show an ontogenetic development, it has been argued that a similar developmental trend should be observed in dichotic listening if the DL test reflects aspects of language function (Geffen & Wale, 1979; Larsen, 1984, 1989).

This question is related further to the more general question of whether brain laterality is subject to ontogenetic development (e.g., Lenneberg, 1967). In general, the assumption is that there should be an increase in right ear advantage (REA) with increasing age, thus reflecting an increase in left-hemispheric specialization for language with age (e.g., Kraft, 1984; Neufeld, 1976). The idea that lateralization is absent at birth and gradually develops over age was defended by Lenneberg (1967) and by Brown and Jaffe (1975). However, very few empirical studies have supported this view. Kraft (1984) found increasing ear advantages in children from 4 years of age. Similarly, Satz, Bakker, Teunissen, Goebel, and Van der Vlugt (1975) found an increase in REA between 9 and 11 years, although no such difference was found among the younger age groups studied.

These studies were exceptions: a clear majority of studies failed to reveal an increase in ear advantage with age. The typical finding has been that a REA can be observed in children as young as 3 years (Ingram, 1975; Piazza, 1977) and that the magnitude of the REA does not change across age (Hynd & Obrzut, 1977; Kinsbourne & Hiscock, 1977; Knox & Kimura, 1970; Van Duyne, Gariguolo, & Gonter, 1984).

However, another typical finding has been that the *overall level of performance* (i.e., overall more correct reports) increases with age. A few studies also reported a *decrease* in ear advantage with increasing age (Larsen, 1984; Simmons & Baltaxe, 1974). Larsen argued that a decrease in ear advantage with increasing age may be observed only when children with a right ear advantage are separated statistically from children with a left, or no, ear advantage.

The question of development of ear advantage may be illustrated with the following cross-sectional study from our laboratory (Asbjørmen et al., 1991). Children aged 5, 8, and 11 years were studied with consonant-vowel (CV) syllables with our standard technique (a more detailed description of the technique is reviewed later). The children were tested under three different recall conditions: free report, where they were allowed to allocate attention between channels and report the item that they heard; forced-right report, in which they attended to and reported only what they heard in the right ear; and forced-left report, in which they attended to and reported only what they heard in the left ear.

The results showed a significant difference in number of overall correct reports, with the 5-year-old children reporting overall fewer correct items. No difference was observed in overall performance between the 8 and 11 year olds. The REA effect was more marked during the second half of the test, particularly for the younger children, indicating a delayed learning effect in younger compared to older children.

Finally, both the 5 and 8 year olds showed a REA despite instructions to attend to and report only from the *left* ear. Thus the ability to shift attention to the ear ipsilateral to the language-dominant hemisphere is reduced in younger children. Hugdahl and B. Andersson (1987) argued that the inability to block out a REA in younger children by attending to the left ear is related to literacy. They found that whereas preliterate children (and particularly boys) could not shift ear advantage with instructions, literate children (as well as adults) could do this easily (see also Hugdahl & L. Andersson, 1986; Obrzut, Hynd, Obrzut, & Pirozzolo, 1981).

Summarizing the studies related to age differences in magnitude of ear advantages, Kinsbourne and Hiscock reflect the current state of what is known: "The question of ontogenetic changes in the ear advantage is not closed, but the best answer at present is that the right-ear advantage does not increase with increasing age" (1981, p. 151).

Methods and Theoretical Assumptions

Dichotic listening means literally listening to two different auditory messages at the same time, one in each ear. The method of dichotic listening was introduced into cognitive psychology by Broadbent in the early 1950s in a study of selective attention in air traffic controllers (Broadbent, 1954). An air traffic controller faces the problem of handling different flight bearings that are received at about the same time. Broadbent developed an experimental analogue by having subjects listen to different messages that arrived in each ear. Broadbent, however, never hypothesized that the phenomenon of selective reports found in his subjects was due to the different processing capacities in the right and left hemispheres.

Kimura (1961a, 1961b) was the first investigator to use the DL technique for the study of laterality and hemispheric asymmetry. In the first of her papers (Kimura, 1961a), she found that patients with epilepsy who were to undergo neurosurgery differed in the frequency of correct reports of speech sounds from the right and left ears, depending on whether they had language localized to the left or right hemisphere. Language lateralization had been established in these patients prior to the DL test through the Sodium Amytal procedure (Wada & Rasmussen, 1960). Specifically, Kimura (1961a) found that patients with left-hemisphere language were more correct in recall of the right ear items, whereas patients with right-hemisphere language were more correct in recall of left ear items. This was corroborated in her second study on normal subjects where all showed a REA (1961b).

Furthermore, others were able to replicate the original findings (e.g., Bryden, 1963), and it was shown that the REA effect also could be obtained in children (Kimura, 1963). Today, the REA effect is probably one of the more robust empirical phenomena coming out of psychological laboratories. The number of published papers on dichotic listening in neuropsychology and cognitive psychology has grown considerably (i.e., there are probably as many as several hundred) in the time that has passed since Kimura's original contribution (see Hugdahl, 1988, for an entire volume devoted to dichotic listening).

Mechanisms Behind the REA Effect

The most frequent explanation for the REA effect in dichotic listening is the so-called structural model (Kimura, 1967). This model assumes that the way dichotic listening is related to brain asymmetry and laterality is through suppression of the ipsilateral auditory pathways and enhancement of the contralateral pathways from the ear to the primary auditory cortex. However, although it has been shown that the contralateral auditory brain regions seem to be more activated during both monaural and dichotic stimulations (Connnolly, 1985; Majkowski, Bochenek, Bochenek, Knapik-Fijalkowska, & Kopek, 1971; Maximilian, 1982; Rosenzweig, 1954), this does not prove that dichotic listening is related to brain asymmetry primarily through the contralateral projections from the ear to the temporal cortex. Further, is not clear if suppression of the ipsilateral pathways takes place at subcortical or cortical levels (cf. Zaidel, 1983).

Kimura (1967) postulated that the REA seen in most right-handed subjects in a DL situation was caused by several interacting factors. First, it was assumed that the auditory input to the contralateral hemisphere was more strongly represented than the ipsilateral input. Second, it was postulated that one hemisphere (the left hemisphere for most individuals) is specialized, or dominant, for the processing of language stimuli. Third, because the information that is routed through the ipsilateral pathways is suppressed, or blocked, by the contralateral information, the ipsilateral information has to cross the corpus callosum to reach the language processing center in the dominant left hemisphere. As a consequence, the REA will reflect either superior processing of the contralateral right ear

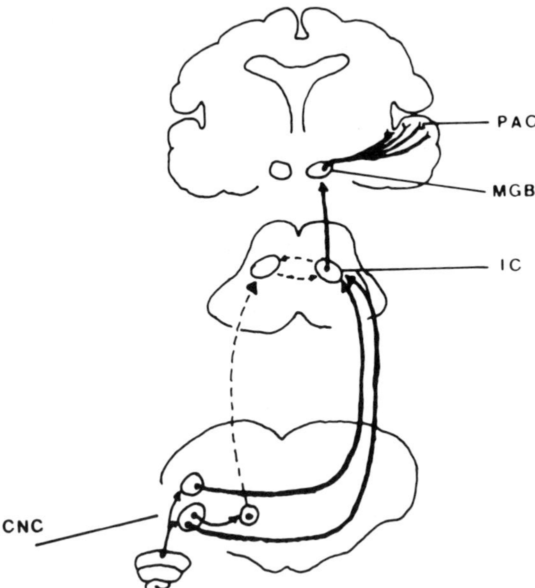

Fig. 5.1. Outline of auditory projections showing the preponderance of the contralateral projections from the cochlea to the temporal auditory cortex. *Key*: CNC, Cochlear nucleus; IC, Inferior colliculus; MGB, Medial geniculate body; PAC, Primary auditory cortex.

pathways or inferior processing of the ipsilateral left ear pathways due to their transcallosal transmission or to the interaction between these factors (see Bradshaw & Nettleton, 1988, for further discussion).

The predominance of the contralateral pathways from the cochlea in the ear to the temporal cortex may be an effect of stronger projection of the second-order neurons to the inferior colliculus on the contralateral than on the ipsilateral side (Brodal, 1981). Thus the pathways *to* the inferior colliculus are larger from the contralateral ear, whereas the pathways ascending *from* the colliculi are greater on the ipsilateral side, favoring an ultimate representation of the *contralateral* ear in the auditory cortex. This is illustrated in Figure 5.1.

The structural model gained empirical support from two classic papers (Milner, Taylor, & Sperry, 1968; Sparks & Geschwind, 1968). Both papers reported a remarkable finding in patients with a sectioned corpus callosum (splitting the brain). In all instances, there was a complete or near-complete extinction in the left ear channel when the right and left ears were stimulated simultaneously with dichotic presentations.

Sparks and Geschwind (1968) reasoned that auditory signals from the left ear, having reached the auditory cortex of the right hemisphere through the more preponderant contralateral pathways, could not be transmitted to the left hemisphere for processing and oral report. Their logic was that in order to get an oral report of the left ear (right-hemisphere) input, the signal should travel from the right auditory cortex, via the corpus callosum, to the language-dominant left-hemisphere region. Consequently, damage to the pathway anywhere along this route should yield extinction of the left ear input. Similarly, lesions in the language-specialized auditory regions of the left hemisphere also should disrupt the outflow from the corpus callosum, and thus produce a left ear extinction as well.

An Attentional Interpretation

As argued by Bradshaw and Nettleton (1988), a crucial test of the structural model is whether ear asymmetries can be obtained with monaural stimulation. Several studies have reported a right ear preference for monaurally presented verbal stimuli (Blackstock, 1978; Palmer, 1964). Furthermore, Bakker (1969, 1970) found that children showed better recall of right ear input compared to left under monaural presentation.

On the basis of these findings, Bradshaw and Nettleton (1988) argued that the traditional dichotic listening paradigm was not necessary in order to generate ear asymmetries. Instead, they suggested that it was the perceived position of a sound source, rather than ear of entry, that determines behavioral asymmetries (see also Bertelsen, 1982). Bradshaw and his colleagues showed a REA by arranging loudspeakers in the room so that they were hidden from the listener (Pierson, Bradshaw, & Nettleton, 1983). They found that when lateralized *visual* cues misled subjects as to the true, nonlateralized source of the auditory signal, it was the *apparent* localization of the source that determined the laterality effect. If the source appeared to come from the right side of space, performance was superior.

A similar view has been proposed by Geffen and Quinn (1984; see also Clark, Geffen, & Geffen, 1988). In their review of ear advantages in DL they concluded that there was strong support for the view that sounds presented in one-half of space are processed quantitatively better in the contralateral hemisphere. Furthermore, they argued that by voluntary direction of attention, the inherent perceptual asymmetry may be overcome.

Another alternative explanation of the REA phenomenon in dichotic listening is the attentional model proposed by Kinsbourne (1970, 1973). Kinsbourne's main argument was that anticipation of a verbal stimulus "primes" the language-specialized (left) hemisphere, thereby increasing its arousal. This anticipation also directs attention to the stimulus source contralateral to the language hemisphere (i.e., to the right ear). Further, priming effects may be more important in children, especially in free report situations (Hiscock & Decter, 1988).

Other data suggest, however, that attentional priming is probably not the sole explanation for the REA in dichotic listening, and especially not in children (Hugdahl & Andersson, 1986), but that both structural and attentional factors contribute to the observed REA. Furthermore, lateral eye movements do not seriously confound the REA. Asbjørnsen, Hugdahl, and Hynd (1990) instructed subjects to fixate their gaze to the left, right, or straight ahead while they at the same time received dichotic presentations of CV syllables. The results showed no differences between eye movement conditions, with a REA in all three conditions.

Dichotic Listening Paradigms

The dichotic listening technique is basically simple. Two different messages are presented at the same time, one in each ear, and the subject, or patient, is requested to repeat in one way or another what was heard. In the early studies (Bryden, 1963; Kimura, 1961a,b; Satz, Achenbach, Pattishall, & Fennell, 1967), lists of numbers were used with blocks of three or four pairs of numbers presented in fairly rapid succession. The subject then had to recall as many items as possible after each block. Later studies used another approach where the subject makes the recall after each stimulus pair is presented on a trial-by-trial basis, with presentation rates between 2 and 5 seconds (e.g., Hugdahl & B. Andersson, 1987; Hugdahl & L. Andersson, 1986).

A problem with the "block technique" is that subjects were left free to adopt different strategies when attending and reporting what they heard. For example, some subjects may have reported what they heard in one ear first, and then what they heard in the other ear. As argued by Bryden (1988), this had the effect that the items reported from the second ear had to be retained in short-term memory longer than the items from the first reported ear, with the result that they were not reported as accurately as items from the first ear.

The use of numbers with the block technique was seriously challenged when Studdert-Kennedy and Shankweiler published their now classic paper in 1970. Studdert-Kennedy and Shankweiler used simple consonant-vowel-consonant (CVC) syllables that were presented in pairs, one to each ear. Within each stimulus pair, only one element was different (i.e., the initial consonant, the vowel, or the final consonant). Studdert-Kennedy and Shankweiler reported reliable REAs in normal adults, with the effect being most pronounced for the consonants, especially for first consonants. No laterality effect was observed for the vowels.

The difficulty of obtaining the REA for vowels also was reported by Hugdahl and L. Andersson (1984), and it has been argued that this might reflect the specialization of the language-dominant hemisphere for the processing of rapidly changing auditory stimuli (e.g., the rapid formant transitions seen in the stop consonants) (Schwartz & Tallal, 1980). Nonetheless, REAs have been obtained for vowels (e.g., Darwin, 1971; Spellacy & Blumstein, 1970).

After the success of the approach pioneered by Studdert-Kennedy and Shankweiler (1970), most researchers adopted this technique, by using only a single consonant together with a single vowel (i.e., CV syllables). This technique also was adopted for studies in children. For example, Obrzut, Boliek, and Obrzut (1986) compared CV syllables, words, and speech stimuli in a dichotic listening task with 10-year-old children. They concluded that CV syllables yielded the most reliable ear advantages and that findings were not distorted easily by attention and strategy factors. Today, the most frequently used dichotic stimuli are the six stop consonants /b/, /d/, /g/, /p/, /t/, /k/ used together with the vowel /a/ to produce CVs such as /ba/, /da/, /pa/.

The Free-Report Paradigm

The most common DL paradigm is the free-report CV syllables paradigm. In the free-report paradigm, subjects are requested to listen to both inputs and try to report both items in the pair as accurately as possible. Thus the subject is free to allocate attention between ears and may also adopt different strategies in the order of report. As argued by Bryden (1988), however, there is some evidence that second choices are no better than guesses and therefore only single correct trials should be scored. Alternatively, subjects should be instructed to always report only *one* item on each trial regardless of whether they perceive one or two items. The experimenter then calculates the number of correct reports from the right and left ear inputs.

My colleagues and I have found over the years that instructing the subject to report only one item is to be preferred, especially when dealing with children and with neurological patients (e.g., Hugdahl, Andersson, et al., 1990; Hugdahl, Wester, & Asbjørnsen, 1990a,b). Another reason for using single-item reports is that the DL situation, although simple on the surface, may easily elicit a feeling of distress from the subject if too much is demanded from him or her. The use of instructions to report only single items also has the advantage that data are not lost as easily as when two items are requested.

A standard dichotic tape frequently used by my colleagues and I consists of three different randomizations of all combinations of the six basic CVs. This yields 36 trials in each randomization, including homonyms (e.g., /ba–ba/) as control trials, with a total of 108 trials. A pause for 30 seconds occurs after each randomization of 36 trials.

Figure 5.2 presents typical results from right-handed adults and children in a free-report CV paradigm. Usually, adults have between 60% and

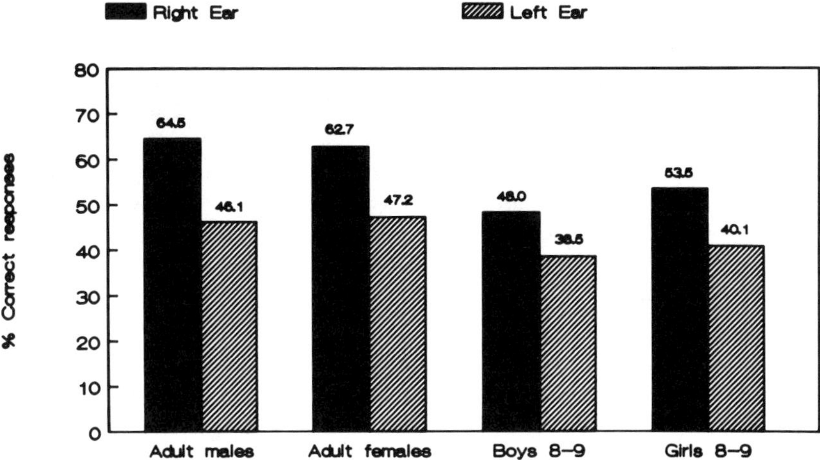

Fig. 5.2. Percentage of correct reports from right and left ear in adults and children, males and females, boys and girls. Data pooled from three different experiments.

80% correct reports from the right ear and between 40% and 60% correct from the left ear. Thus the typical REA in adults under free report is about 20%. Children between 8 and 9 years of age perform overall with about a 10% reduction in both correct right and left ear reports compared to adults. The data in Figure 5.2 are pooled from a series of experiments (Hugdahl & B. Andersson, 1987; Hugdahl & L. Andersson, 1986)

The Forced-Attention Paradigm

Some investigators have suggested that the REA effect may be brought about by a bias to attend selectively to the right side of space (e.g., Geffen & Wale, 1979; Kinsbourne, 1970; Treisman & Geffen, 1968). When subjects are left free to report the items in a DL situation, they may choose the order in which they report, especially when double-correct items are requested. They also may attend differentially to the right and left ear input (Bryden, Munhall, & Allard, 1983; Hugdahl & L. Andersson, 1986). Further, it could be argued that right-handed subjects find it easier to focus attention on items from the right ear rather than those from the left.

The forced-attention paradigm controls for strategy and attentional effects by having the subjects attend to and report only the *right* ear input in one-third of the trials, to attend to and report only the *left* ear input in another third of the trials, and to be free to allocate attention in either way in a final third of the trials (Bryden et al., 1983; Hugdahl & L. Andersson, 1986). The presentation order is counterbalanced across subjects.

By comparing the number of correct reports from *the left ear* during forced attention to the *right ear*, with the number of correct reports from the *right ear* during forced attention to the *left ear*, an "attention-free" asymmetry score may be obtained. The reason for this is that items reported from the nonattended ear during forced attention to the opposite ear should reflect intrusions from the contralateral hemisphere. Thus if a REA exists for nonattended items during forced attention, which is comparable to the REA obtained during nonforced attention, then selective attention alone cannot explain the REA effect. In the Somatic Psychology laboratory, a new set of instructions about attention to the right or left ear is given after each series of 36 CV trials using the standard DL tape. Thus the score for each subject usually is based on 30 pairs of CV presentations within each attentional instruction (excluding the 6 homonymes).

The forced-attention paradigm has proved to be quite important when studying the development of cognitive functions such as reading and its interaction with laterality (B. Andersson & Hugdahl, 1987; Hugdahl & B. Andersson, 1987). Hugdahl and L. Andersson (1986) compared right-handed adults and 8- to 9-year-old children in a forced-attention test. A significant REA was observed in both adults and children during the free-report instruction and during the forced-right instruction. However, during the forced-left instruction, the children *still reported more correct items from the right ear*. This was particularly evident for the boys. Thus the study by Hugdahl and L. Andersson showed that the REA cannot be disrupted in children of that age by explicit instructions to attend only to the *left ear* (cf. Obrzut, Obrzut, Bryden, & Bartels, 1985). Similar findings were reported by Hiscock and Kinsbourne (1980) and by Sexton and Geffen (1979). The results for the children from the Hugdahl and L. Andersson study are presented in Figure 5.3.

An interesting implication of these findings is that whereas attentional ability is subject to age-related development, cerebral asymmetry apparently is not. The finding that asymmetry already is present in infancy was demonstrated by Witelson and Pallie (1973) and by Molfese and Molfese (1979). The findings by Hugdahl and L. Andersson (1986) thus imply not only that attention should be controlled in studies of laterality, but also that laterality should be controlled in studies of attention.

In a follow-up study, Andersson and Hugdahl (1987) showed that whereas 8-year-old children could not shift attention to the left ear input during the dichotic test, 9 year olds could do so when the same children were retested exactly 1 year later. Thus a developmental shift was observed for attention, but nor for laterality. This is seen in Figure 5.4.

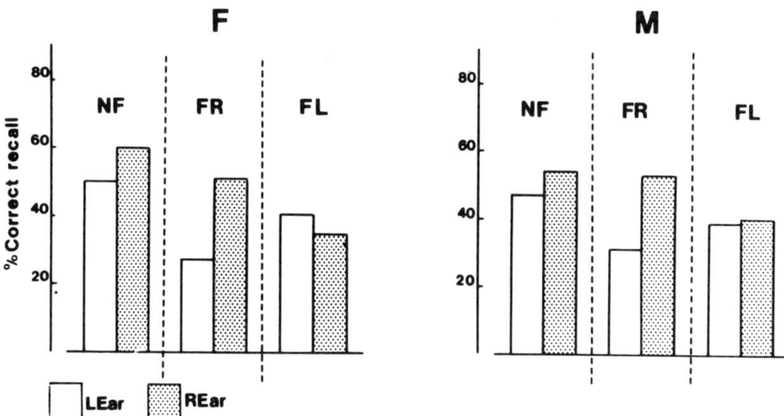

Fig. 5.3. Percentage of correct reports during nonforced (NF), forced-right (FR), and forced-left (FL) attentional instructions. *Key*: F, females (girls); M, males (boys). From "The Forced-Attention Paradigm in Dichotic Listening to CV-Syllables: A Comparison Between Adults and Children" by K. Hugdahl and L. Andersson, 1986, *Cortex*, *22*, p. 424. Copyright 1986 by Cortex. Reprinted by permission.

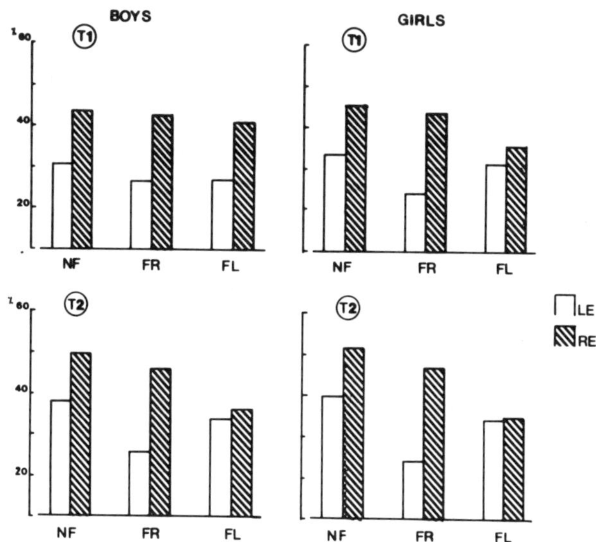

Fig. 5.4. Percentage of correct reports to CV syllables during nonforced (NF), forced-right (FR), and forced-left (FL) attentional instructions. *Key*: T1, first test at the age of 8; T2, second test at the age of 9; LE, left ear correct; RE, right ear correct. From "Effects of Sex, Age, and Forced Attention on Dichotic Listening in Children: A Longitudinal Study" by B. Andersson and K. Hugdahl, 1987, *Developmental Neuropsychology*, *3*, p. 196. Copyright 1987 by Developmental Neuropsychology. Reprinted by permission.

The Fused-Rhymed Paradigm

A third paradigm often used in DL studies is the fused-rhymed test, or fused dichotic listening test, developed by Halwes and Wexler (Halwes, 1969; Wexler & Halwes, 1983). The fused-rhymed paradigm is based on improving the stimulus parameters rather than altering the instructions to the subject. Wexler and Halwes (1983) used rhyming pairs of words that were selected so that the two sounds fuse into a coherent perceptual unit. The logic behind the "fused" test is that in order to secure suppression of ipsilateral input, overlap between the members of each stimulus pair should be maximized. This is achieved by using stimulus pairs that are identical except for one distinguishing component (e.g., /aba/ and /aka/) (see also Wexler, 1988).

An interesting finding is that although subjects claim that they hear only "one stimulus in the middle of the head," they nevertheless report this to be the right ear stimulus item in most cases. The fused-rhymed paradigm yields robust and reliable REAs comparable to the REAs obtained with the CV paradigms (Wexler & Halwes, 1983).

The Target-Monitoring Paradigm

The target-monitoring paradigm (e.g., Clark et al., 1988; Geffen & Caudrey, 1981; Geffen & Sexton, 1978) requires the subject to monitor series of word pairs, with one word from each pair being presented to the left and the other to the right ear. Whenever a predesignated "target" word is heard, the subject is instructed to indicate manually (e.g., by pressing a button) or orally that he or she has detected the target. Thus subjects are requested to monitor the stream of stimulus input closely in order to detect the targets accurately.

The targets occur an equal number of times in the right and left ear. A typical monitoring test consists of CVC syllables, and a target word in one ear may be opposed by semantically or phonemically similar words. The target-monitoring paradigm allows for analysis of both accuracy of the right and left ear input and of reaction time whenever a target is detected. Furthermore, it is possible to use the paradigm in child populations that lack expressive language.

The target-monitoring paradigm was used in a study by Bø, Hugdahl, and Marklund (1989) on 11-year-old children with serious speech problems. The dichotic test consisted of three different CVC target words in Norwegian, /"mor"/ (mother), /"ror"/ (row), and /"bor"/ (live), interspersed among series of phonemically similar distractor wods like /"gor"/ and /"lor"/. The children were asked to point at a sheet on which a picture representing the target word was printed whenever they heard the target in the headphones.

The results revealed an increased number of the subjects with a left ear advantage (LEA), and there was also a marked reduction in the magnitude of the REA in those children who showed a REA. Thus the DL target-monitoring technique demonstrated that children with serious speech problems were inferior to normal children in REA magnitude and in the number of subjects with a REA.

Preparation of Dichotic Tapes

Traditionally, dichotic stimuli are presented from a stereo tape recorder where the two items of each pair of stimuli are recorded separately on the left and right channels of the tape. With the increasing use of personal computers (PCs) in both research and clinical work, it is now possible, at least in principle, to present the dichotic stimuli directly from the computer using an internal sound chip together with appropriate software and hardware supplies. However, although the dichotic situation appears simple and easy to handle, the preparation of high-quality dichotic tapes is tedious work that requires access to both computer technology and technical skills. The single most important aspect of the preparation of a DL tape is the temporal synchronization between channels (i.e., making sure that the two stimuli of a pair have equal onset times). As Berlin (1977) showed, even such a small asynchrony as 15 ms can be detected by the brain, with this asynchrony being reflected in a change in the reported frequencies between the ears.

Early Tapes

If one considers the limited computer technology available to psychologists in the early 1960s and 1970s, one must be impressed by the power of the dichotic listening method, given that reliable REAs were reported even though some investigators at that time prepared their tapes by recording a list of numbers on one channel, then rewinding the tape and recording a different list on the other channel (see history by Bryden, 1988).

Anyone who has the slightest experience with stereophonic tape recorders knows that it is impossible to listen to one channel and record something different on the other channel at exactly the same time. Thus it is not surprising that the early DL literature was plagued by conflicting results, with some investigators questioning the validity of the DL technique. It is important to realize, however, that despite the poor technical quality of the stimulus tapes, reliable REAs were found in most studies. It is also important to keep in mind the poor technology available for the early students of DL, and especially when comparing results from different laboratories over time.

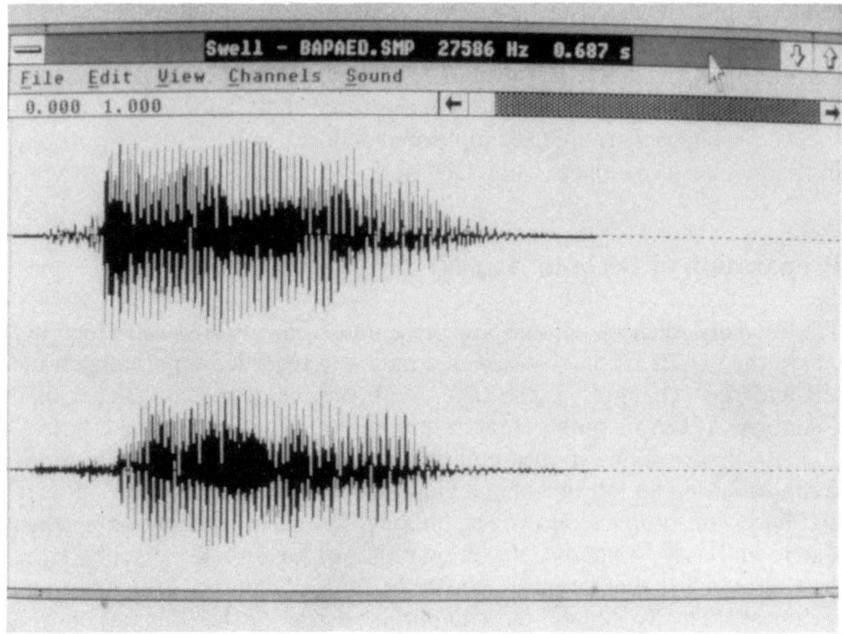

Fig. 5.5. Computer display of the CV syllables /ba/ (upper) and /pa/ (lower) from the PC-based software for aligning dichotic stimuli.

Software Packages

A computer software package called CADDIC (Hugdahl, Nordstrand, & Engstrand, 1986) developed in Bergen in the early 1980s allowed for exact onset and offset alignment of the two stimuli in a pair, as well as exact control of intensity differences between channels. The CADDIC software also allowed for alignment to be performed on either the consonant or vowel onset in a CV pair, or for alignment of both sounds, an aspect of the DL situation often neglected in the literature (see Figure 5.5).

The CADDIC software was developed to be run on a PDP 11/45 machine and thus requires access to a minicomputer laboratory system. With the widespread use of PCs, we developed a new system that runs as an application under Microsoft-Windows on an IBM-AT. This system is easier to use and does not require huge investments in hardware. Figure 5.5 shows an example of a display of the CVs /pa/ and /ba/ from the new software package.

We routinely use natural speech that is digitized at a minimum sampling rate of 10 kHz and fed to the analogue-to-digital (A/D) conversion board

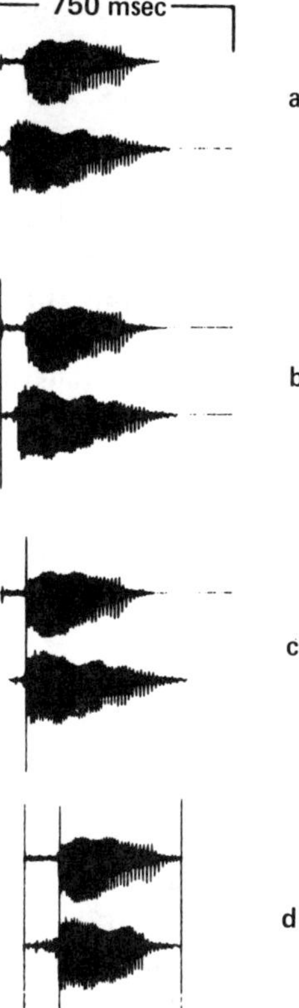

Fig. 5.6. Oscillographic displays of the CV syllables /pa/ (upper) and /ba/ (lower) with different synchronizations (*b–d*). From "A Graphic-Interactive CAD System for Dichotic Stimulus Alignment (CADDIC)" by K. Hugdahl, L. Nordstrand, and O. Engstrand, 1986, *Psykologisk Rapportserie*, 7, No. 3, p. 11. Copyright 1986 by Universitetet i Bergen. Reprinted by permission.

in the computer. Pairs of CVs are displayed on the computer monitor and listened to over loudspeakers; the onset coordinates then are identified for each CV pair. After satisfactory editing for synchronization and intensity, the file containing the series of CVs is fed over a digital-to-analogue (D/A) board back to the tape recorder and recorded on a master tape. Cassette copies can then easily be produced from the master tape.

Figure 5.6 presents an example of the difference between temporal alignment on the *consonant* versus *vowel* segments of a CV pair, with computer displays of the CVs /pa/ above and /ba/ below. Figure 5.6a reveals that the /pa/ onset consists of an abrupt burst of random noise followed by glottal pulsing related to the vowel. The /ba/ sound, on the other hand, shows a relatively weak initial energy release which precedes the release of the glottal pulsing.

As seen in Figure 5.6(b–d) temporal alignment, or synchronization, can be achieved in at least three different ways, each with its own phonetic implications for the perception of the dichotic stimulus pair. In Figure 5.6b, the two syllables are synchronized with respect to the initial energy release in the consonant segment. This means, however, that *the vowel onset will be asynchronous*. This is the most popular way of constructing dichotic tapes, and most studies are probably performed with consonant segment synchronization. In Figure 5.6c, the synchronization criterion is shifted from the initial consonant onset to the vowel segment. However, this has the implication that *the consonant onset will be asynchronous*.

The optimal solution is seen in Figure 5.6d, which shows the combination of initial consonant and secondary vowel alignment criteria; that is, the syllables are aligned *on both the consonant and vowel segments*. In addition, the syllables are equalized for overall duration. Although this procedure seems to be the best solution, it should be kept in mind that the combined alignment slightly changes the "natural" acoustic structure of the original speech records. In my experience, however, this does not seriously alter the perception of the dichotic stimuli and does not affect the REA.

The Dichotic Test Situation

With the development of sophisticated computer programs for the construction of dichotic tapes, minicassette players, like the Sony Walkman, are good enough for *testing*, particularly in natural settings (e.g., the school situation, the clinic). This is probably even more important when dealing with children who otherwise might get frightened by, or exceptionally interested in, all of the technical equipment in the research laboratory.

If instructions to attend to a particular ear are used when testing preschool children, it is advisable to use a prop (e.g., a doll or some other toy) that is held on the targeted side. The experimenter may then instruct the child "to listen *only* to the ear on the same side as the doll." It is also advisable to instruct children that sounds they are about the hear "do not mean anything," and that they simply should repeat what they hear without thinking about what the sounds may mean.

Scoring of Dichotic Responses

Several scoring techniques and statistical procedures are used for examining dichotic results; all have their own characteristics and their own pros and cons. The interested reader may consult Speaks (1988) and Harshman and Lundy (1988) for updated reviews of scoring methods and the statistics of DL scores. Only a summary is provided here.

When considering the more sophisticated theoretical aspects of the different scoring procedures, the beginning student may become confused and unsure about which procedure to use. The best advice is offered by Harshman and Lundy:

Initially, measures of laterality were proposed, at least in part, on empirical and psychological grounds; later, the arguments became entirely formal and mathematical . . . [several authors] . . . attempted to choose the "best" asymmetry index on purely formal grounds, by looking for an index that had desirable mathematical properties. . . . This shift in arguments apparently corresponded to an unstated shift in objectives. These later authors could not find persuasive arguments to indicate which index would best reflect underlying hemispheric asymmetry, and so they concentrated on formal arguments which indicated that their methods optimally quantified surface asymmetry. (1988, pp. 216–217)

Since there appears to be no "best and ultimate" asymmetry index for dichotic scores, my colleagues and I have adopted the approach of staying as close as possible to the raw scores.

The Difference Score

The simplest and probably most frequently used scoring procedure is to calculate the number of correct right and left ear reports separately. These may be converted to percentage-correct scores for each ear with ear advantage expressed as percent right ear minus percent left ear. There may be a right ear advantage, a left ear advantage, or a no ear advantage (NEA) when correct right ear scores equal correct left ear scores. Although simple and easy to use, the difference-score technique has the disadvantage that it does not compensate for differences between subjects in overall levels of accuracy. This is handled by the index score.

The Index Score

The typical index score is calculated as a ratio of the difference between the ears. This is done by dividing the right ear and left ear difference by the total number of correct reports from both ears:

$$\text{index score} = \frac{\text{RE} - \text{LE}}{\text{RE} + \text{LE}} \times 100$$

Thus the index score will vary between +100 (maximum right ear advantage) and −100 (maximum left ear advantage), with zero indicating no ear advantage.

The major advantage with the index score is that it compensates for differences in overall performance (Marshall, Caplan, & Holmes, 1971). Other statistical procedures based on different methods to treat the index-score concept include the phi-coefficient (Kuhn, 1973), lambda-statistics (Bryden & Sprott, 1981), and percent of correct (POC) and percent of errors (POE) techniques (Harshman & Lundy, 1988). These latter methods are not discussed here. However, Hiscock and Decter (1988) argued that any laterality index, including right minus left ear scores, is likely to be biased for age-related asymmetry shifts. Therefore, they warn against uncritical use of laterality indexes in children.

Magnitude Versus Frequency Data

The question of magnitude versus frequency data relates to the issue of "degrees" of laterality and whether such differences can be detected by the DL method. Berlin (1977) argued that dichotic listening could be regarded at best as a correlate of laterality for language, but not as an *index* of the magnitude of laterality. Thus it would be an error to infer that a subject with a 70% REA is "more" left-hemisphere lateralized for language than a subject with a 55% REA. Kinsbourne and Hiscock (1981) further argued that lateralization (in right-handers) probably is an all-or-none phenomenon; that is, *all* subjects showing a REA in a DL test should be regarded as left-hemisphere dominant for language, regardless of individual differences in *the magnitude* of the REA. A different approach was advocated by Harshman and Lundy (1988), who argued, on the basis of data from commissurotomized patients, that laterality is probably *not* an all-or-none phenomenon, but that there are quantitative differences in asymmetry for perceptual and cognitive functions.

One way to approach this problem is to complement magnitude data (whether as difference or index scores) with scatter plots of frequency of subjects showing a particular ear advantage. An important but often neglected question is how many subjects showed more correct reports from the ear that was the better ear in the overall group mean regardless of the magnitude of the advantage. This means applying nonparametric statistics to DL scores, which some investigators have argued sacrifices much of the information in the raw data (e.g., Hiscock & Decter, 1988). Supplementing parametric statistics for group mean data with nonparametric statistics for frequency data, however, actually may enhance the information available in the raw scores. For example, Hugdahl and Franzon (1987) found that although both male and female adults showed a significant REA, with no differences in group means, the male group revealed more homogeneity when frequency data were analyzed. Thus whereas group mean data showed no sex differences, frequency data did.

This can be illustrated as follows. Suppose that a significant mean REA was found in a group of 20 children. This, however, does not tell us *how many* of the 20 children showed a REA (which most clinicians probably are more interested in). A significant group mean REA may be obtained even if a substantial proportion of the children actually showed a LEA, provided that a few of those showing a REA had *very large* REAs, and the LEAs were *small*. Further, an analysis of variance would not treat a LEA as *qualitatively* different from a REA. Theoretically, however, a LEA (regardless of magnitude) should be treated as indicative of a right-hemisphere language specialization, and a REA should be treated as indicative of a left-hemisphere specialization. Thus the qualitative difference between the REA and LEA will not be reflected in quantitative statistical analyses. This may be particularly important when DL is

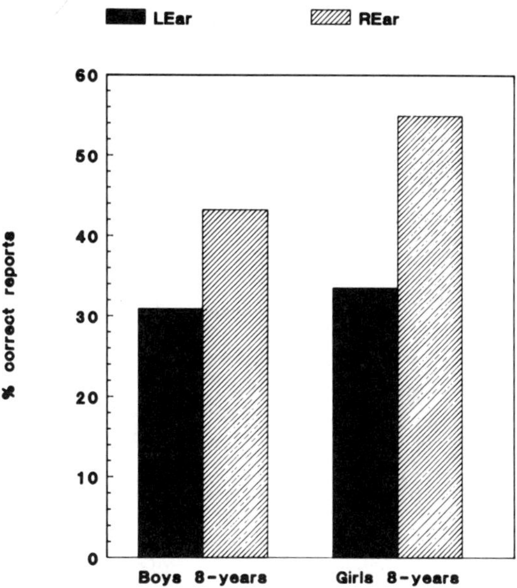

Fig. 5.7. Group mean data showing percentage of correct reports for boys and girls. *Key*: LEar, left ear correct; REar, right ear correct.

used in applied settings for assessments of laterality dominance patterns, for example, with children with seizures where invasive tests cannot be performed for clinical reasons.

By providing information about frequency data, in addition to magnitude data, the clinical significance of the DL technique may also be substantially improved (see Hugdahl & Øst, 1981, for a discussion of statistical versus clinical significance). This is illustrated in Figures 5.7 and 5.8, which show magnitude and frequency data, respectively, during free report for 76 eight-year-old children (38 boys and 38 girls).

As can be seen in Figure 5.7, there was a significant REA for both boys and girls in the magnitude range of 12% to 20%. Looking at the corresponding frequency data, Figure 5.8 shows that only 2 boys had a LEA, whereas 3 boys showed a NEA. A NEA was scored for those subjects that fell on the 45-degree "symmetry line." Thus 86.8% of the boys revealed a REA. The picture was almost the same for the girls, although there were slightly more girls with a LEA; 7 girls showed a LEA, 1 girl a NEA, and 30 (78.9%) revealed a REA. Also seen in Figure 5.8, the variation in degree of ear advantage was larger among the boys than among the girls.

Figure 5.9 shows the relative ear advantage of a 9-year-old left-handed girl with a tumor in the right frontal lobe compared to a group of normal

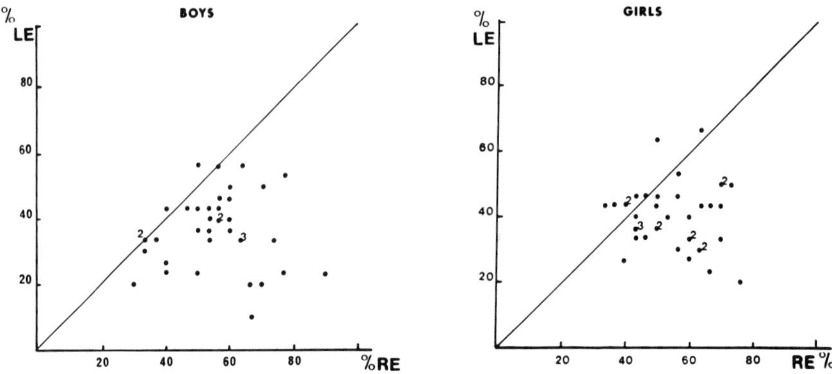

Fig. 5.8. Scattergrams of distributions of boys and girls in the "ear-advantage space." Note the "45-degree symmetry line," which represents no ear advantage. Small numbers inside the scattergram means that more than one subject occupies the same coordinates. Data as in Figure 5.7. *Key*: LE, left ear correct reports; RE, right ear correct reports. From "Effects of Sex, Age, and Forced Attention on Dichotic Listening in Children: A Longitudinal Study" by B. Andersson and K. Hugdahl, 1987, *Developmental Neuropsychology*, *3*, pp. 200, 201. Copyright 1987 by Developmental Neuropsychology. Reprinted by permission.

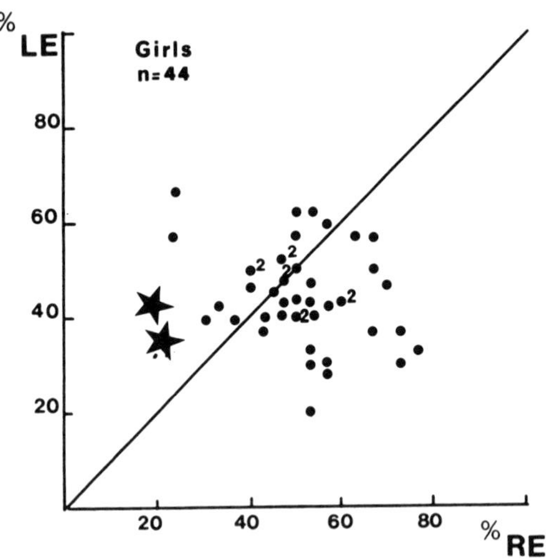

Fig. 5.9. The large "stars" in the scattergram show the ear advantage for a 9-year-old left-handed girl with a brain tumor relative to 44 normal intact 8- and 9-year-old left-handed girls. *Key*: LE, left ear correct reports; RE, right ear correct reports.

left-handed children. The patient was to receive an operation for the tumor, but because she showed language difficulties it was suspected that she might be right-hemisphere dominant for language. An invasive test with Sodium Amytal was not recommended for clinical reasons, and it was decided to perform a dichotic listening test.

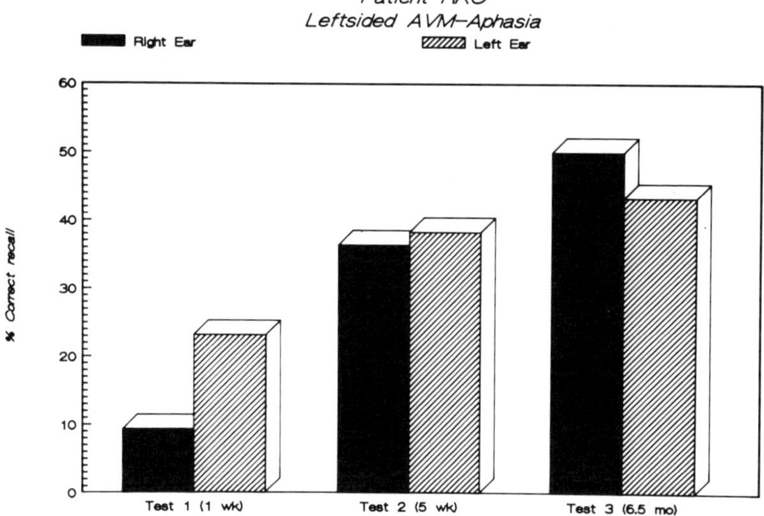

Fig. 5.10. Percentage of correct reports during a free-report condition for an 18-year-old aphasic male after a left-sided subcortical hemorrhage. First DL test after 1 week, second test after 5 weeks, and third test after 612 months.

The patient was tested twice with about a 3 hour interval between the two tests. The results are seen in Figure 5.9 as stars in the scattergram, together with data from 44 intact 8- and 9-year-old left-handed girls. The patient deviated from the majority of left-handed girls, with her results serving to indicate right-hemisphere dominance for language.

The significance of the DL procedure as a clinical alternative to invasive methods is obvious in this example, with a consistent DL response profile related to localization of language functions. It should be noted that DL also taps asymmetry for *reception* of verbal *input*, whereas Sodium Amytal basically taps asymmetry for *production* of verbal *output*.

Another example of the clinical use of DL is seen in Figure 5.10 (data from Hugdahl, Wester, & Asbjørnsen, in 1990b). The patient was an 18-year-old aphasic male who suffered from a subcortical hemorrhage in the left frontoparietal region with involvement of Broca's area. The patient was tested three times with dichotic listening, 1 week after the acute hemorrhage, 5 weeks after, and again about 6 months after the hemorrhage. At the first testing he could not speak at all but understood well. At the second testing he uttered one-syllable words and could answer "yes" and "no" to questions. At the third testing, he could speak whole sentences, although slowly and not fluently. His dichotic listening performance showed an almost perfect correspondence to his speech recovery. As seen in Figure 5.10, on the first DL testing he showed a LEA, which changed to a NEA on the second testing, and then to a REA on the third testing. His overall performance also was markedly reduced on the first testing but improved on the following assessments.

Once again, the DL procedure allowed a detailed analysis of recovery of both input and output language capacity not revealed in standard clinical evaluations. Theoretically, it could further be speculated that the LEA observed during the acute aphasic phase either reflected limited right-hemisphere language input processing capacity (caused by the *contralateral* left ear input) or preserved left-hemisphere language functions (caused by the *ipsilateral* left ear input).

Validity

One way to assess the validity of the dichotic listening test in children is to examine the proportion of right- and left-handed children who show REA and LEA, respectively. Because invasive tests for language laterality typically show that more than 95% of right-handed adults have left-hemisphere language representation (Rasmussen & Milner, 1977; Strauss, Gaddes, & Wada, 1987; Wada & Rasmussen, 1969), one should expect the DL task to yield a REA in at least 95% of the right-handed population (cf. Hiscock & Decter, 1988).

Most studies report proportions that vary from 65% to about 90%, depending on the type of test given and the type of scoring procedure used (Bryden & Allard, 1978; Hiscock & Kinsbourne, 1977). A majority of the findings are gathered on adults, however, and researchers usually do not take differences in the magnitude of the REA between individuals into account. For example, two studies may show equal REA proportions, although the distribution of individuals across the magnitude spectrum may vary substantially between the same studies.

There is also the ambiguous issue of how to treat individuals who score close to the 45-degree symmetry line (as in Figure 5.8), but on opposite sides. For example, does a 3% REA represent a *qualitatively* different brain organization than a 3% LEA? In this chapter, it is argued that a REA, however small, should be treated as reflecting left-hemisphere processing, and a LEA, however small, should be treated as reflecting right-hemisphere processing.

Figure 5.11 presents frequency data for 126 left-handed and 152 right-handed 8- and 9-year-old children. A significant REA was obtained in both groups, and the magnitude of the REA was similar for both right-handers (17.1%) and left-handers (18.2%). However, the distributions of number of subjects showing a particular ear advantage and the variability within the groups were quite different for the right- and left-handed children. Thus whereas 84.2% of the right-handed children showed a REA, this was true only for 65.0% of the left-handed children.

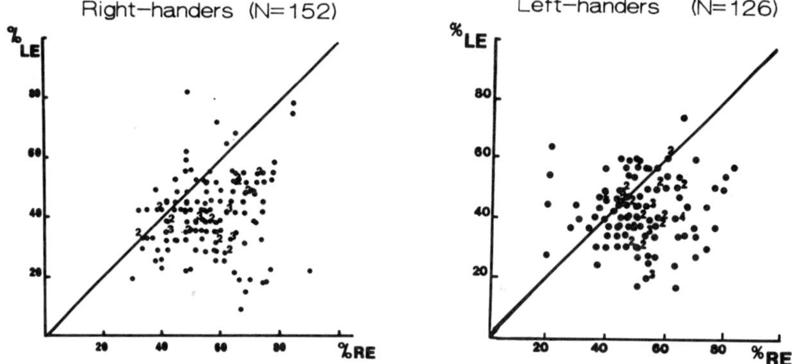

Fig. 5.11. Sample data pooled from several experiments in our laboratory showing scattergrams of distributions of right- and left-handed children in the "ear-advantage space." Note 45-degree symmetry line. Numbers inside the scattergrams means that more than one subject occupies the same coordinates. *Key*: LE, left ear correct reports; RE, right ear correct reports.

In comparing these data with the 95% left-hemisphere language dominant (for right-handers) and 70% right-hemisphere language dominant (for left-handers) figures reported from studies with Sodium Amytal (e.g., Rasmussen & Milner, 1977), the DL results in Figure 5.11 of 84.2% and 65.0% underestimate the actual figures by 11% and 5% for left- and right-hemisphere language representation, respectively. However, this does not necesssarily mean that DL is less accurate as a technique. First of all, it should be kept in mind that DL is a noninvasive technique, and that there is rarely *any* neuropsychological test (or any test of cognitive functions for that matter) that can show a 100% correspondence with invasive data. Also, the discrepant figures may reflect differences between children and adults.

Second, invasive techniques mainly monitor expressive language functions, whereas DL, to a large extent, is a test of verbal recognition and perception (Bradshaw & Nettleton, 1981) and may also reflect subcortical functions (cf. Hugdahl, Wester, & Asbjørnsen, 1990a; Mateer & Ojemann, 1983). Furthermore, Porter and Berlin (1975) suggested that perception of CV syllables in DL taps basic phonetic functions rather than more complex semantic functions.

Third, not all Sodium Amytal studies have shown the same consistent results. Strauss et al. (1987) found that only 7 out of 12 left-handed patients had speech represented in the left hemisphere (i.e., 58.3%) compared to other Amytal studies showing 70% of all left-handers to be left-hemisphere dominant (i.e., a discrepancy of 11.7%). This suggests that differences in procedures between laboratories doing Sodium Amytal studies also may influence the comparative results.

Reliability

Measures of reliability of DL scores in children vary between .70 and .90. Bakker, Van der Vlugt, and Claushuis (1978) studied children up to the fifth grade and found 1 week test–retest correlations to vary between .70 and .87. Harper and Kraft (1986) and Kraft (1985) reported figures between .78 and .87 and between .88 and .93, respectively, for similar tests. The variation in figures usually stems from differences in the index scores used, the kind of stimuli used, and the age levels investigated. Looking specifically at reliability for CV syllables, Koomar and Cermak (1981) found test–retest reliability to be .89 for normal children and .88 for learning-disabled children.

Reliability coefficients that are obtained over short time periods (e.g., 1 week) may not necessarily reflect stability over longer periods. For example, Teng (1981) found large differences in correlation coefficients for adults studied over a 6 month period. Andersson and Hugdahl (1987) compared the number of children who maintained or switched their ear advantage when tested first at the age of 8 and later at the age of 9. The results showed that only 17% of the boys switched ear advantage over a 1 year period, whereas 83% maintained their ear advantage. The corresponding figures for the girls were 28% who switched ear advantage and 72% who maintained their ear advantage.

Hiscock and Decter (1988) also argued that DL scores do not necessarily correlate with other measures of laterality, like the visual half-field (VHF) test (see also Searleman, 1980). Instead of simply dismissing DL as a nonvalid technique, it may be that DL and VHF tap different aspects of brain laterality. It is probably a mistake to assume that the advantage for a hemisphere for two different tasks should reflect the *same* underlying dichotomy (e.g., verbal-visuospatial). As argued by Hellige (1990), the search for a fundamental dichotomy that defines all information processing differences between the hemispheres has so far been without success, and there is even reason to question whether success is possible.

Sex Differences

It generally is believed that females have a more diffuse, or less lateralized, cerebral organization of language (Bryden, 1979; McGlone, 1980), although Kimura (1985) questions this. Reviewing the literature on sex differences in dichotic listening in adults, Bryden (1988) concluded that he had not found any study where a greater proportion of REA was found in females. The problem is, however, that not all studies show a greater proportion of REA in males. Thus the conclusion is that there probably are sex differences in dichotic listening performance, although they are small and of marginal significance (Bryden, 1988).

In looking at sex differences in DL performance in children, data consistently failed to demonstrate differences between girls and boys (both right- and left-handed) in ear advantage magnitudes under free-report conditions (B. Andersson & Hugdahl, 1987; Hugdahl & B. Andersson, 1989a). However, the *variability* is often greater among girls. This has been particularly true for left-handed children in our studies. Clear sex differences have emerged, however, when girls and boys were compared in the forced-attention paradigm (i.e., when instructed to pay attention and to report only from one ear).

Conclusions

This chapter has reviewed the use of dichotic listening to CV syllables in children, focusing on practical procedures and paradigms. Several methods for presenting dichotic stimuli were presented along with guidelines on how to prepare dichotic tapes and conduct testing procedures. Normative data on both free-report and forced-attention procedures were given for different age groups, for both right- and left-handers, and for males and females. Examples from neurological patients also were illustrated.

A major argument of this chapter is that although proportions of subjects with a particular ear advantage do not perfectly match the proportions of subjects found to have a particular language dominance when tested with invasive techniques (e.g., Sodium Amytal), the DL method still has enough power (compared to most other noninvasive methods of neuropsychological investigation) to be applied in clinical settings. The REA found in DL is a surprisingly robust *empirical* phenomenon, although the theoretical explanations of it differ among investigators. Seen in this perspective, DL is a useful tool for examining brain–behavior relationships in children, particularly those involving higher cortical functioning like language, attention, and memory.

Further work is needed to examine issues of convergent and divergent validity when comparing DL with other measures of laterality. However, as previously argued, the lack of correlation between tachistoscopic VHF tests and DL is not a critical issue because they probably measure different capacities within the same hemisphere. Furthermore, DL also reflects differences in attentional capacity *between* the hemispheres (e.g., Broadbent, 1954) with implications for short-term memory (Christianson, Nilsson, & Silfvenius, 1987). Thus low intercorrelations between tests do not necessarily reflect low validity for the tests; they may simply not be measuring the same unitary phenomenon. The notion that hemispheric asymmetry is a global cognitive faculty in itself, independent of other cognitive functions, should be replaced by a more fine-grained analysis including asymmetries for different cognitive functions. This has been often ignored in the literature of hemispheric asymmetry, probably because the bulk of the *empirical* evidence has come from studies of perceptual asymmetry with very few studies related to, for example, learning and memory. Moreover, although studies of shifts of brain asymmetry patterns in children with learning *disorders* are abundant (see, e.g., Obrzut & Boliek, 1988, for review), there are very few, if any, studies of asymmetry related to *normal* learning, or shifts in asymmetry related to the *normal* acquisition of the reading skill (see Hugdahl & B. Andersson, 1989b, for an exception). I hope that this chapter has elucidated some of these questions and that future research may also address issues not usually studied today.

Acknowledgments. The present research was supported by the Norwegian Council for Research in the Social Sciences (NAVF-RSF).

References

Andersson, B., & Hugdahl, K. (1987). Effects of sex, age, and forced attention on dichotic listening in children: A longitudinal study. *Developmental Neuropsychology*, *3*, 191–206.

Asbjørnsen, A., Hugdahl, K., & Hynd, G. W. (1990). The effects of head and eye-turns on the right ear advantage in dichotic listening. *Brain and Language*, *39*, 447–458.

Asbjørnsen, A., Hugdahl, K., Christiansen, S.Å., Säisa, J., & Lyytinen, H. (1991) Effects of training and biased attention on dichotic listening, performance in children. *Reports from the Department of Psychology*, *University of Stockholm*, #735.

Bakker, D. J. (1969). Ear-asymmetry with monaural stimulation: Task influences. *Cortex*, *5*, 36–42.

Bakker, D. J. (1970). Ear-asymmetry with monaural stimulation: Relations to lateral dominance and lateral awareness. *Neuropsychologia*, *8*, 103.

Bakker, D. J., Van der Vlugt, H., & Claushuis, M. (1978). The reliability of dichotic ear asymmetry in normal children. *Neuropsychologia*, *16*, 753–757.

Berlin, C. I. (1977). Hemispheric asymmetry in auditory tasks. In S. Harnad, R. W. Doty, L. Goldstein, J. Jaynes, & G. Krauthamer (Eds.), *Lateralization in the nervous system* (pp. 303–332). New York: Academic Press.

Berlin, C. I., Hughes, L. F., Lowe-Bell, S. S., & Berlin, H. L. (1973) Dichotic right ear advantage in children 5 to 13. *Cortex*, *9*, 394–402.

Bertelsen, P. (1982). Lateral differences in normal man and lateralization of brain function. *International Journal of Psychology*, *17*, 173–210.

Blackstock, E. G. (1978). Cerebral asymmetry and the development of early infantile autism. *Journal of Autism and Childhood Schizophrenia*, *8*, 339–353.

Bø, O., Hugdahl, K., & Marklund, E. (1989). Dichotic listening in children with serious language problems. *Perceptual and Motor Skills*, *68*, 1291–1301.

Bradshaw, J. L., & Nettleton, N. C. (1981). The nature of hemispheric specialization in man. *Behavior and Brain Sciences*, *4*, 51–92.

Bradshaw, J. L., & Nettleton, N. C. (1988). Monaural asymmetries. In K. Hugdahl (Ed.), *Handbook of dichotic listening: Theory, methods and research* (pp. 45–70). Chichester, U.K.: Wiley.

Broadbent, D. E. (1954). The role of auditory localization in attention and memory span. *Journal of Experimental Psychology*, *47*, 129–133.

Brodal, A. (1981). *Neurological anatomy* (3rd ed.). New York: Oxford University Press.

Brown, J. W., & Jaffe, J. (1975). Hypothesis on cerebral dominance. *Neuropsychologia*, *13*, 107–110.

Bryden, M. P. (1963). Ear preference in auditory perception. *Journal of Experimental Psychology*, *65*, 103–105.

Bryden, M. P. (1979). Evidence for sex-related differences in cerebral organization. In M. Witting & A. C. Petersen (Eds.), *Sex-related differences in cognitive functioning: Developmental issues* (pp. 1–44). New York: Academic Press.

Bryden, M. P. (1988). An overview of the dichotic listening procedure and its relation to cerebral organization. In K. Hugdahl (Ed.), *Handbook of dichotic listening: Theory, methods and research* (pp. 1–44). Chichester, U.K.:Wiley.

Bryden, M. P., & Allard, F. A. (1978). Do auditory perceptual asymmetries develop? *Cortex*, *17*, 313–318.

Bryden, M. P., Munhall, K., & Allard, F. (1983). Attentional biases and the right-ear effect in dichotic listening. *Brain and Language*, *18*, 236–248.

Bryden, M. P., & Sprott, D. A. (1981), Statistical determination of degree of laterality. *Neuropsychologia*, *19*, 571–581.

Christianson, S. Å., Nilsson, L. G., & Silfvenius, H. (1987). Initial memory deficits and subsequent recovery in two cases of head trauma. *Scandinavian Journal of Psychology*, *28*, 267–280.

Clark, C. R., Geffen, L. B., & Geffen, G. (1988). Invariant properties of auditory perceptual asymmetry assessed by dichotic monitoring. In K. Hugdahl (Ed.), *Handbook of dichotic listening: Theory, methods and research* (pp. 71–84). Chichester, U.K.: Wiley.

Connolly, J. F. (1985). Stability of pathway-hemispheric differences in the auditory event-related potential (ERP) to monaural stimulation. *Psychophysiology*, *22*, 87–96.

Darwin, C. J. (1971). Ear differences in the recall of fricatives and vowels. *Quarterly Journal of Experimental Psychology*, *23*, 46–62.

Geffen, G., & Caudrey, D. (1981). Reliability and validity of the dichotic monitoring test for language laterality. *Neuropsychologia*, *19*, 413–423.

Geffen, G., & Quinn, K. (1984). Hemispheric specialization and ear advantages in processing speech. *Psychological Bulletin*, *96*, 273–291.

Geffen, G., & Sexton, M. A. (1978). The development of auditory strategies of attention. *Developmental Psychology*, *14*, 11–17.

Geffen, G., & Wale, J. (1979). The development of selective listening and hemispheric asymmetry. *Developmental Psychology*, *15*, 138–146.

Halwes, T. G. (1969). *Effects of dichotic fusion on the perception of speech. Status report on speech research*. New Haven, CT.: Haskins Laboratories.

Harper, L. V., & Kraft, R. H. (1986). Lateralization of receptive language in preschoolers: Test–retest reliability in a dichotic listening task. *Developmental Psychology*, *22*, 553–556.

Harshman, R. A., & Lundy, M. E. (1988). Can dichotic listening measure "degree of lateralization"? In K. Hugdahl (Ed.), *Handbook of dichotic listening: Theory, methods and research* (pp. 215–282). Chichester, U.K.: Wiley.

Hellige, J. B. (1990). Hemispheric asymmetry. *Annual Review of Psychology*, *41*, 55–80.

Hiscock, M., & Decter, M. H. (1988). Dichotic listening in children. In K. Hugdahl (Ed.), *Handbook of dichotic listening: Theory, methods and research* (pp. 431–477). Chichester, U.K.: Wiley.

Hiscock, M., & Kinsbourne, M. (1977). Selective listening asymmetry in preschool children. *Developmental Psychology*, *13*, 217–224.

Hiscock, M., & Kinsbourne, M. (1980). Asymmetries of selective listening and attention switching in children. *Developmental Psychology*, *16*, 70–82.

Hugdahl, K. (1988). (Ed.). *Handbook of dichotic listening: Theory, methods and research*. Chichester, U.K.: Wiley.

Hugdahl, K., & Andersson, B. (1987). Dichotic listening and reading acquisition in children: A one-year follow-up. *Developmental Neuropsychology*, *9*, 631–649.

Hugdahl, K., & Andersson, B. (1989a). Dichotic listening in 126 left-handed children: Ear advantages, familial sinistrality and sex differences. *Neuropsychologia*, *27*, 999–1006.

Hugdahl, K., & Andersson, B. (1989b). Visual half-field tests of lateralized letter presentations: Differences between preliterate and literate children. *International Journal of Neuroscience*, *44*, 215–226.

Hugdahl, K., & Andersson, L. (1984). A dichotic listening study of differences in cerebral organization in dextral and sinistral subjects, *Cortex*, *20*, 135–141.

Hugdahl, K., & Andersson, L. (1986). The forced-attention paradigm in dichotic listening to CV-syllables: A comparison between adults and children. *Cortex*, *22*, 417–432.

Hugdahl, K., Andersson, L., Asbjørnsen, A., & Dalen, K. (1990). Dichotic listening, forced attention, and brain asymmetry in right- and left-handed children. *Journal of Clinical and Experimental Neuropsychology*, *12*, 539–548.

Hugdahl, K., Ellertsen, B., Waaler, P. E., & Kløve, H. (1989). Left and right-handed dyslexic boys: An empirical test of some assumptions of the Geschwind-Behan hypothesis. *Neuropsychologia*, *27*, 223–231.

Hugdahl, K., & Franzon, M. (1987). Dichotic listening performance to CVs between versus within groups. *Scandinavian Journal of Psychology*, *28*, 26–34.

Hugdahl, K., Nordstrand, L., & Engstrand, O. (1986). A graphic-interactive CAD system for dichotic stimulus alignment (CADDIC). *Psykologisk Rapportserie* (Universitetet i Bergen), 7, No. 3.

Hugdahl, K., & Øst, L. G. (1981). On the difference between statistical and clinical significance. *Behavioral Assessment*, *3*, 289–295.

Hugdahl, K., Synnevaag, B., & Satz, P. (1990). Immune and auto-immune diseases in dyslexic children. *Neuropsychologia*, *28*, 673–679.

Hugdahl, K., Wester, K., & Asbjørnsen, A. (1990a). The role of the left and right thalamus in language asymmetry: Dichotic listening in Parkinson-patients undergoing stereotactic thalamotomy. *Brain and Language*, *39*, 1–13.

Hugdahl, K., Wester, K., & Asbjønsen, A. (1990b). Dichotic listening in an aphasic male patient after a subcortical hemhorrage in the left fronto-parietal region. *International Journal of Neuroscience*, *54*, 139–146.

Hynd, G. W., & Obrzut, J. E. (1977). Effects of grade level and sex on the magnitude of the dichotic ear advantage. *Neuropsychologia*, *15*, 689–692.

Ingram, D. (1975). Cerebral speech lateralization in young children. *Neuropsychologia*, *13*, 103–105.

Kimura, D. (1961a). Some effects of temporal lobe damage on auditory perception. *Canadian Journal of Psychology*, *15*, 156–165.

Kimura, D. (1961b). Cerebral dominance and the perception of verbal stimuli. *Canadian Journal of Psychology*, *15*, 166–171.

Kimura, D. (1963). Speech lateralization in young children as determined by an auditory test. *Journal of Comparative and Physiological Psychology*, *56*, 899–902.

Kimura, D. (1967). Functional asymmetry of the brain in dichotic listening. *Cortex*, *3*, 163–168.

Kimura, D. (1985, November). Male brain, female brain: The hidden difference. *Psychology Today*.

Kinsbourne, M. (1970). The cerebral basis of lateral asymmetries in attention. *Acta Psychologica*, *33*, 193–201.

Kinsbourne, M. (1973). The control of attention by interaction between the cerebral hemispheres. In S. Kornblum (Ed.), *Attention and performance* (Vol. 4, pp. 239–256). New York: Academic Press.

Kinsbourne, M., & Hiscock, M. (1977). Does cerebral dominance develop? In S. J. Segalowitz & F. A. Gruber (Eds.), *Language development and neurological theory* (pp. 46–68). New York: Academic Press.

Kinsbourne, M., & Hiscock, M. (1981). Cerebral lateralization and cognitive development. In G. W. Hynd & J. E. Obrzut (Eds.), *Neuropsychological assessment and the school-age child* (pp. 12–32). New York: Grune & Stratton.

Knox, C., & Kimura, D. (1970). Cerebral processing of nonverbal sounds in boys and girls. *Neuropsychologia*, *8*, 227–237.

Koomar, J. A., & Cermak, S. A. (1981). Reliability of dichotic listening using two stimuli formats with normal and learning-disabled children. *American Journal of Occupational Therapy*, *35*, 456–463.

Kraft, R. H. (1984). Lateral specialization and verbal/spatial ability in preschool children: Age, sex, and familial handedness differences. *Neuropsychologia*, *22*, 319–335.

Kraft, R. H. (1985). Laterality and school achievement: Interactions between familial handedness and assessed laterality. *Perceptual and Motor Skills*, *61*, 1147–1156.

Kuhn, G. M. (1973). The phi-coefficient as an index of ear differences in dichotic listening. *Cortex*, *9*, 450–457.

Larsen, S. (1984). Developmental changes in the pattern of ear asymmetry as revealed by a dichotic listening task. *Cortex*, *20*, 5–17.

Larsen, S. (1989). *Laesning og cerebral integration.* (trans. *Reading and cerebral integration*) Copenhagen: Gyldendal.

Lenneberg, E. (1967). *Biological foundations of language*. New York: Wiley.

Majkowski, J., Bochenek, Z., Bochenek, W., Knapik-Fijalkowska, D., & Kopek, J. (1971). Latency of average evoked potentials to contralateral and ipsilateral stimulation in normal subjects. *Brain Research*, *25*, 416–419.

Marshall, J. C., Caplan, D., & Holmes, J. M. (1971). The measure of laterality. *Neuropsychologia*, *13*, 315–321.

Mateer, C., & Ojemann, G. A. (1983). Thalamic mechanisms in language and memory. In S. J. Segalowitz (Ed.), *Language function and brain organization* (pp. 171–189). New York: Academic Press.

Maximilian, V. A. (1982). Cortical blood flow asymmetry during monaural verbal stimulation. *Brain and Language*, *15*, 1–11.

McGlone, J. (1980). Sex differences on human brain asymmetry: A critical survey. *Behavioral and Brain Sciences*, *3*, 215–227.

Milner, B., Taylor, L., & Sperry, R. W. (1968). Lateralized suppression of dichotically presented digits after commissural section in man. *Science*, *161*, 184–186.

Molfese, D. L., & Molfese, V. J. (1979). Hemisphere and stimulus differences as reflected in the cortical responses of newborn infants to speech stimuli. *Developmental Psychology*, *15*, 505–511.

Neufeld, G. A. (1976). The relationship of speech-sound discrimination to the development of ear asymmetries in grade-school children. *Dissertation Abstracts International*, *36*, 3653–3654.

Obrzut, J. E., & Boliek, C. A. (1988). Dichotic listening: Evidence from learning and reading disabled children. In K. Hugdahl (Ed.), *Handbook of dichotic listening: Theory, methods and research* (pp. 475–530). Chichester, U.K.: Wiley.

Obrzut, J. E., Boliek, C. A., & Obrzut, A. (1986). The effect of stimulus type and directed attention on dichotic listening with children. *Journal of Experimental Child Psychology*, *41*, 198–209.

Obrzut, J. E., Hynd, G. W., Obrzut, A., & Pirozzolo, F. J. (1981). Effect of directed attention on cerebral asymmetries in normal and learning-disabled children. *Developmental Psychology*, *17*, 118–125.

Obrzut, J. E., Obrzut, A., Bryden, M. P., & Bartels, S. G. (1985). Information processing and speech lateralization in learning-disabled children. *Brain and Language*, *25*, 87–101.

Palmer, R. D. (1964). Cerebral dominance and auditory asymmetry. *Journal of Psychology*, *58*, 157–167.

Piazza, D. M. (1977). Cerebral lateralization in young children as measured by dichotic listening and finger tapping tasks. *Neuropsychologia*, *15*, 417–425.

Pierson, J. M., Bradshaw, J. L., & Nettleton, N. C. (1983). Head and body space to left and right, front and rear: I. Unidirectional competitive auditory stimulation. *Neuropsychologia*, *21*, 463–473.

Porter, R. J., & Berlin, C. I. (1975). On interpreting developmental changes in the dichotic right-ear advantage. *Brain and Language*, *2*, 186–200.

Rasmussen, T., & Milner, B. (1977). The role of early left-brain injury in determining lateralization of cerebral speech function. *Annals of the New York Academy of Sciences*, *299*, 355–369.

Rosenzweig, M. R. (1954). Cortical correlates of auditory localization and of related perceptual phenomena. *Journal of Comparative and Physiological Psychology*, *47*, 264–276.

Satz, P., Achenbach, K., Patishall, E., & Fennell, E. (1967). Order of report, ear asymmetry and handedness in dichotic listening. *Cortex*, *1*, 377–396.

Satz, P., Bakker, D. J., Teunissen, J., Goebel, R., Van der Vlugt, H. (1975). Developmental parameters of the ear asymmetry: A multivariate approach. *Brain and Language*, *2*, 171–185.

Schwartz, J., & Tallal, P. (1980). Rate of acoustic change may underlie hemispheric specialization for speech perception. *Science*, *207*, 1380–1381.
Searleman, A. (1980). Subject variables and cerebral organization for language. *Cortex*, *16*, 239–254.
Sexton, M. A., & Geffen, G. (1979). The development of three strategies of attention in dichotic monitoring. *Developmental Psychology*, *15*, 299–310.
Simmons, J. Q., & Baltaxe, C. (1974). Dichotic listening in gifted and normal children. In *Cerebral dominance* (Brain Information Service Conference Report 34). Los Angeles: University of California.
Sparks, R., & Geschwind, N. (1968). Dichotic listening in man after section of neocortical commissures. *Cortex*, *4*, 3–16.
Speaks, C. E. (1988). Statistical properties of dichotic listening scores. In K. Hugdahl (Ed.), *Handbook of dichotic listening: Theory, methods and research* (pp. 185–214). Chichester, U.K.: Wiley.
Spellacy, F., & Blumstein, S. E. (1970). The influence of language set on ear preference in phoneme recognition. *Cortex*, *6*, 430–439.
Springer, S. P. (1986). Dichotic listening. In H. J. Hannay (Ed.), *Experimental techniques in human neuropsychology* (pp. 138–166). New York: Oxford University Press.
Strauss, E., Gaddes, W. H., & Wada, J. A. (1987). Performance on a free-recall verbal dichotic listening task and cerebral speech dominance determined by the carotid amytal test. *Neuropsychologia*, *25*, 747–753.
Studdert-Kennedy, M., & Shankweiler, D. P. (1970). Hemispheric specialization for speech perception. *Journal of the Acoustical Society of America*, *48*, 579–594.
Teng, E. L. (1981). Dichotic ear difference is a poor index for the functional asymmetry between the cerebral hemispheres. *Neuropsychologia*, *19*, 235–240.
Treisman, A. M., & Geffen, G. (1968). Selective attention and cerebral dominance in perceiving and responding to speech messages. *Quarterly Journal of Experimental Psychology*, *20*, 139–150.
Van Duyne, H. J., Gargiulo, R. M., & Gonter, M. A. (1984). The effect of word presentation rate on monaural and dichotic ear-asymmetry in school age children. *International Journal of Clinical Neuropsychology*, *6*, 175–183.
Wada, J., & Rasmussen, T. (1960). Intracarotid injection of sodium amytal for the lateralization of cerebral speech dominance. *Journal of Neurology*, *21*, 399–405.
Wexler, B. E. (1988). Dichotic presentation as a method for single hemisphere stimulation studies. In K. Hugdahl (Ed.), *Handbook of dichotic listening: Theory, methods and research* (pp. 85–116). Chichester, U.K.: Wiley.
Wexler, B. E., & Halwes, T. (1983). Increasing the power of dichotic methods: The fused rhymed words test. *Neuropsychologia*, *21*, 59–66.
Witelson, S. F., & Pallie, W. (1973). Left-hemisphere specialization for language in the human newborn: Neuroanatomic evidence of asymmetry. *Brain*, *96*, 641–646.
Zaidel, E. (1983). Disconnection syndrome as a model for laterality in the normal brain. In J. B. Hellige (Ed.), *Cerebral hemisphere asymmetry* (pp. 95–151). New York: Praeger.

CHAPTER 6

Cognitive Rehabilitation Following Traumatic Brain Injury in Children

MARK YLVISAKER, SHIRLEY F. SZEKERES, and PATRICK HARTWICK

Traumatic brain injury (TBI) does not initially appear to be a useful category for purposes of designing rehabilitation or special education programs. Unlike other disability and special education categories in childhood, traumatic brain injury identifies a *cause* of potential disability, not the disability itself. Given variation in the nature and location of the brain injury, virtually any area or combination of areas of functioning can be affected. Furthermore, severity can range from injuries producing death or persistent coma to injuries from which children recover quickly and completely. Finally, a disproportionately large number of children with head injury have a pretrauma history of learning or behavior problems (Brown, Chadwick, Shaffer, Rutter, & Traub, 1981; Rutter, 1981; Rutter, Chadwick, Shaffer, & Brown, 1980). There is enormous diversity within this group of children.

Why, then, have we chosen this clinical population for a discussion of cognitive intervention? A full answer to this question would include discussion of (1) deficits frequently seen in these children, particularly cognitive deficits and their pathophysiologic basis, and (2) ways in which central tendencies in this group are similar to and different from central tendencies in other disability groups.

Cognitive Deficits

Regardless of the site of impact in severe closed head trauma, the brain is vulnerable to several distinct types of injury. Primary impact damage, including contusion, laceration, and axon shearing, predictably occurs in areas where the brain abuts bony prominences on the interior surface of the skull (Pang, 1985). This explains the high incidence of orbital-frontal and bilateral anterior temporal lobe injuries. In addition, differential movement of brain tissue within the skull produces widespread, diffuse axonal injury. Together, these lesions help to account for the frequency with which one observes disorders of self-regulatory function ("executive system" deficits), impaired memory/new learning, disorganized thinking and acting, slowed information processing, reduced attentional control, concrete and egocentric thinking, impaired judgment, and social disinhibition.

Substantial coup and contrecoup lesions, intracranial bleeds, or focal damage related to skull penetration or depressed skull fracture may add a set of deficits related specifically to the site of impact or hemorrhage. Thus specific aphasic syndromes (e.g., Broca's aphasia, Wernicke's aphasia) and academic deficit syndromes (e.g., dyslexia, dyscalculia) may occur, but they are not common. Following traumatic brain injury, most school-age children recover gross physical function, surface language function (i.e., phonologic, morphologic, and syntactic components), and overlearned academic skills (reading recognition, spelling, and basic arithmetic), although perhaps at a lower level than before the injury.

Comparison with Other Disability Categories

Many children with mild to moderate injuries, as measured by early indices such as length of unconsciousness, duration of posttraumatic amnesia, Glasgow Coma Scale (GCS), or Children's Coma Scale, recover completely (Chadwick, Rutter, Brown, Shaffer, & Traub, 1981). Cognitive functioning and behavioral self-control may be depressed for a few days to a few weeks, and therefore these children may require a careful transition from hospital to participation in a full academic and social schedule. However, this is not the group under consideration in this chapter.

Children with injuries that appear initially to be very severe (GCS of 8 or less, coma of several days or more) often experience a remarkable recovery of physical and global intellectual functioning but are frequently left with residual information processing and self-regulatory deficits that may resemble those of children with developmental learning disabilities and attention deficits. Children in both groups tend to evidence uneven cognitive and academic profiles; have greater difficulty learning new information and skills than would be predicted by results of IQ tests; process information slowly and inefficiently; have difficulty with attentional control, impulse control, and strategic thinking; may lack age-appropriate social skills; and appear to profit from similar teaching techniques, including task analysis, precision teaching, multisensory teaching, teaching to strengths, applied behavior analysis, social skills instruction, strategy instruction, and a focus on metacognition.

There are, however, important differences between "typical" children with TBI and "typical" children with learning disabilities. Early in their recovery, head injured children have a much greater degree of overall confusion, disorientation, and episodic memory impairment than their learning disabled peers. Furthermore, their profiles may be more "gappy," showing surprising islands of preserved knowledge or skill as well as unexpected gaps at lower levels of functioning than would be expected in the case of a child whose learning disability has been present from birth. Because of the predictably good return of pretraumatically overlearned information and skills, children in the late stages of recovery from TBI may have little difficulty with surface language skills and core academic skills (e.g., reading recognition, spelling, writing, calculating) that learning disabled children may be struggling to acquire. This means that the curriculum in a learning disabilities classroom may strikingly miss the needs of the head injured child, despite many similarities in cognitive profiles among the two groups of children. Furthermore, for several months or even years after the injury, the child with TBI may continue to recover neurologically, albeit at a sharply decreasing rate. This instability argues against giving the child with TBI a firm disability label that might interfere with flexible readjustment of the child's program as recovery occurs.

Some children who are functionally more compromised by their injury may have intelligence test results that place them in a category with children with mental retardation. Indeed, the learning efficiency of these two groups of children may be similar. However, here again there are important differences. Significantly impaired children with TBI may perform surprisingly well on pretraumatically overlearned tasks and in familiar environments. Due to neurological recovery, their prognosis for functional improvement may be superior to that of retarded children. Furthermore, they may retain global adaptive behavior skills, have a well-preserved sense of humor and sense for social reality, and typically retain a self-image that renders placement in a class for children with mental retardation emotionally challenging and/or degrading.

Traumatic brain injury in children thus presents a challenge to professionals in the fields of rehabilitation and special education. Those who would take comfort in the time-honored hypothesis that the young brain possesses a remarkable ability to recover from early injury (i.e., the plasticity hypothesis, or Kennard Principle) should be sobered by the finding that infants have perhaps the worst outcome of any age group following traumatic brain injury (Raimondi & Hirschauer, 1984) and that young children appear to do no better—and maybe worse—than adolescents and young adults in cognitive and psychosocial outcome (Brink, Garret, Hale, Woo-Sam, & Nickel, 1970; Chadwick, Rutter, Brown, et al., 1981; Klonoff, Low, & Clark, 1977; Levin, Eisenberg, Wigg, & Kobayashi, 1982). Even carefully controlled animal experiments have shown that youth may confer a disadvantage rather than an advantage in recovery from certain types of lesion, including bilateral frontal lobe lesions, which are very common in closed head injury (Kolb, 1989).

Severely injured children, therefore, may require special services. However, they may fail to qualify for these services because eligibility criteria have evolved to address the needs of children whose disability exists from birth, and because special education decision makers often interpret criteria narrowly, lacking an understanding of traumatic brain injury or its subsequent recovery process.

Cognitive Rehabilitation

Understood most broadly, rehabilitation includes many types of intervention designed to promote recovery and help people achieve their goals following injury or other disabling event. Cognitive rehabilitation, then, includes a variety of interventions delivered by a variety of professionals designed to promote recovery and to help individuals overcome barriers posed by cognitive impairments. In contrast, if understood as a specialized service designed to return cognitive functioning to its preinjury state by means of targeted cognitive exercises, cognitive rehabilitation is highly controversial and probably no easier to defend than the historically discredited attempts to improve general cognitive and academic functioning by means of perceptual and perceptual-motor exercises (Kavale & Mattson, 1983).

A more fruitful approach to cognitive rehabilitation takes improved performance of real-world tasks as its goal, as opposed to improved "cognition." The deliverers of this service include all professionals who address task performance that may be affected by cognitive weakness. The general modalities include engineering the environment to promote improved performance, selecting learning tasks and instructional strategies that fit the cognitive characteristics of the child, equipping children with their own strategies to compensate for deficits that will not go away, increasing children's base of general information and organizational schemes so that incoming information is easier to process, and heightening children's understanding of their needs so that they become more active participants in solving the many problems caused by the injury and consequent deficits.

In this chapter, we focus on organization and learning—and discuss them together—because of the significance and pervasiveness of these dimensions of cognition for children, the frequency of their impairment following traumatic brain injury, and their essential interconnectedness. Furthermore, all professionals in rehabilitation and special education settings, not just those whose scope of practice includes cognitive rehabilitation or academic instruction, profit from an understanding of these dimensions of development (and recovery), because they affect the acquisition of any knowledge or skill.

In normally developing young children, and in older children early in recovery from brain injury, learning is largely a by-product of engagement in activities that are interesting to the child and that have a meaningful organizational structure. Our discussion of early development therefore focuses on involuntary (or incidental) learning and ways of enhancing involuntary learning through the organization of the task and the development of organizational schemes that enhance the child's learning and adaptive behavior.

Later in child development—and later in recovery following brain injury—children acquire greater understanding of and voluntary control over their cognitive behavior and are able to use strategies in a deliberate manner to learn more efficiently (i.e., deliberate or voluntary learning). Strategies to compensate for cognitive deficits are particularly important for children whose recovery is generally good but who are left with residual impairments that interfere with academic and social success. The second part of this discussion therefore explores the domain of compensatory learning strategies. Because the deliberate use of strategies to improve performance presupposes substantial development—or recovery—of "metacognitive" or "executive" functioning, this chapter ends with a discussion of procedures designed to improve children's functioning in this critical area.

Organization and Learning: Early Development

Normal Development of Memory/Learning

An understanding of normal cognitive development serves several purposes in pediatric rehabilitation. First, normal development imposes limits on treatment goals. For example, it is developmentally inappropriate to expect a 3 year old, or an older child with significant cognitive weakness, to monitor task demands and learning capability and then deliberately use strategies to improve performance. Second, normal development suggests treatment goals and their sequence. For example, knowing that preschoolers perform especially well in learning tasks that include an interesting *thematic* organization of the information to be remembered suggests that reacquisition (or acquisition) of meaningful childhood scripts may be an important goal in cognitive rehabilitation.

Caution must be attached, however, to the use of a developmental template in setting goals. Some developmental targets may be blocked by the nature and severity of the child's brain injury. In other cases, children may need to acquire cognitive skills that would not be expected of their cognitively intact peers. Adolescents with cognitive impairment and a new set of academic and social problems, for example, may need to be more acutely aware of their strengths and limitations and more effective in problem solving than peers whose automatic cognitive behavior serves them adequately.

Furthermore, caution must be exercised because traumatic brain injury can result in widely disparate profiles of ability and need; applying a developmental sequence of goals and remedial activities in a rigid "curricular" fashion blinds one to individual differences that must be the primary driving force in planning rehabilitation and special education. For example, an adolescent with a severe visual scanning deficit but good language recovery may profit from a "top-down" approach to the visual deficit, including exercises composing paragraphs on a word processor. Familiarity with the keyboard together with the facilitating effect of the language that the student has just composed may make this type of exercise most useful in promoting more efficient visual scanning, even though the exercise is at a much higher level developmentally than the target deficit.

Third, an understanding of normal development guides professionals in selecting an appropriate manner of instruction. Developmentally young children, for example, benefit most from learning tasks that are concrete and personally meaningful, that are organized in a way that fits the child's organizational thinking, and that have target information vividly highlighted.

What Develops?

Schneider and Pressley (1989) discussed the development of memory/learning under four interconnected headings: short-term memory, memory strategies, metamemory, and knowledge base. According to these investigators, these are the primary developing components of memory. As such, they are critical areas for exploration in planning treatment.

Short-Term Memory

This is the temporary "holding space" in which information is attended to and either discarded or operated on in some way and transferred to more permanent storage. Short-term memory span is limited, but it does develop with age (7 plus or minus 2 units of information in normal adults). Schneider and Pressley concluded from their review of a large number of developmental studies that improvement in memory span in children is largely a result of increases in *functional* capacity rather than *structural* capacity. Increases in functional capacity are due to several factors, including increased *speed* of information processing, increasingly *automatic* processing of information, and the use of *strategies* to organize information. Kail (1984) emphasized these aspects of efficiency as critical in memory development. Speed, automaticity, and strategies are all based, in part, on growth of the child's knowledge base.

Memory Strategies

Schneider and Pressley (1989) emphasized the important distinction between unconscious, automatic information processing activities and those activities carried out by conscious effort. The word "strategy" has been used for both concepts. In this discussion, we identify strategies as deliberately applied procedures designed to accomplish some goal. Memory strategies may be used at the time of *encoding* (i.e., taking information in) or *retrieval*. Later in this chapter we explore the development of strategies and discuss Siegler's (1986) important point that strategies evolve as part of broader cognitive changes, including improvements in self-monitoring, understanding of tasks and goals, and general problem-solving behavior.

Metamemory

Metamemory evolves as part of metacognitive development, which plays a powerful role in the development of strategic behavior. This is of particular importance in closed head injury, given the frequency of frontal lobe injury and consequent executive system deficits. Metacognition comprises an understanding of one's cognitive functioning and factors that influence cognitive abilities (i.e., the "static" component) and self-regulatory control over cognitive behavior (i.e., the "dynamic" component), including deliberate attempts to remember or to solve problems (Ylvisaker & Szekeres, 1989). Metamemory specifically includes knowledge about persons (e.g., that remembering and forgetting are identifiable experiences distinguishable from thinking, dreaming, etc.), tasks (e.g., that some memory tasks are more difficult than others), and strategies (e.g., that there are things that can be done to make a memory task easier), (Flavell, 1985).

During the early preschool years, children evidence little understanding of their memory (except to reject memory tasks that are too difficult) and seem to use the word "remember" to refer to finding something, whether they knew it was there or not (Brown, 1978; Flavell, 1979; Kail, 1984). By age 5, there seems to be an understanding that memory presupposes previous exposure. Subsequent development includes increasing awareness of one's own ability to remember. Preschool children, for example, can predict their performance in jumping, but they vastly overestimate remembering ability (Kail, 1984). In general, young children tend to be unaware of their lack of knowledge and the implications for performing a task (Markham, 1977).

Furthermore, young children and children with limited cognitive skills generally fail to identify tasks that require special effort (Flavell, 1979; Loper, 1980; Perlmutter & Meyers, 1979). Increasing ability to discriminate task demands is illustrated by the acquisition in the early school years of an understanding that relatedness and familiarity of the material makes remembering easier (Kail, 1984). Finally, although kindergartners may use simple concrete strategies (e.g., placing skates in front of the door in response to "Remember to take your skates"; Flavell, 1985), it is not until much later that children acquire an understanding of the role of strategies in varied learning tasks (Kail, 1984; Siegler, 1986). For example, Kreutzer, Leonard, and Flavell (1975) found that fifth graders are much more likely than younger children to understand their role in learning and to appreciate the need to be actively engaged in the process.

Knowledge Base

The knowledge base includes information, concepts, schemes, and words as well as their interrelations or connections. Because knowledge of an object or event includes organizational components (i.e., its network of connections to other objects or events), knowledge and organization are hard to separate. As knowledge increases, information is more easily organized, integrated, and elaborated (Bjorklund, 1985; Chi, 1978). Similarly, as organizing ability improves, knowledge is more easily acquired.

Involuntary and Deliberate Learning/Memory

Involuntary learning is that which occurs as a by-product of the individual's engagement in personally meaningful activities, in which the goal is not to learn something, but is rather intrinsic to the activity. It also has been referred to as "incidental" learning; however, this term is used ambiguously in the literature and may cause confusion (Postman, 1964). Deliberate (voluntary) learning, on the other hand, is characterized by an intent to learn or remember some information; that is, the goal of the activity is the abstract goal of learning or remembering something (Brown, 1975, 1979; Smirnov, 1973). Studying for an exam, trying to learn or remember words or stories presented in a memory test, and thinking about a person's name during an introduction are examples of deliberate learning. It is unfortunate that most memory tests are deliberate learning tasks; that is, the explicit goal of the task is to remember what is presented. This is particularly unfortunate in the case of young children whose primary mode of learning is involuntary.

Soviet psychologists have consistently emphasized the importance of involuntary memory in children and the transition from involuntary to deliberate learning (Smirnov, 1973). Because young children lack an understanding of learning strategies, instructing them "to learn" or "to remember" cannot be expected to result in any productive activity designed to enhance memory. On the contrary, active engagement in personally meaningful tasks promotes deeper processing of the information and increases the likelihood of encoding, storage, and future recall.

Schneider and Pressley (1989) summarized the results of a series of experiments designed to compare young children's learning within deliberate and involuntary learning tasks. A common finding among preschool children was that deliberate learning instructions (i.e., orienting the child to the task of learning) produced poorer recall than instructions that simply oriented the child to an interesting task with no mention of learning or memory (i.e., involuntary learning tasks). In contrast, older children who have recall strategies (e.g., repetition, rehearsal) often perform better in deliberate learning tasks (Istominia, 1977).

The potency of the involuntary learning condition for young children is likely a consequence of the need to process information at some level of depth in order to make it memorable. If clearly oriented to an interesting task that has a meaningful and motivating goal, and that has the target information highlighted within the concrete activity, preschoolers' learning can be extremely efficient. Orienting an individual to the abstract task of *learning* is helpful only if that individual has a repertoire of strategies that can be used to make the information memorable, whether the context of presentation promotes deep processing or not. The "orienting task" is that which is identified by the instructions (Postman & Kruesi, 1977). If the orienting task ensures the child's engagement and attention to the features of the information that are to be remembered, the likelihood of recall is enhanced. For example, asking a child to sort toys by size and color in preparation for playing a game will increase the probability that he will remember the perceptual aspects of the objects.

Therapy or instructional tasks are, in effect, orienting tasks and can be either favorable or antagonistic to learning. Unfortunately, it is common for therapists and teachers to orient impaired young learners to the task of learning despite evidence that orienting tasks that make learning involuntary are far more effective.

Although preschoolers do not initiate memory strategies in laboratory experiments using voluntary memory situations, they do exhibit early deliberate attempts to learn in natural situations (Istominia, 1977). It is therefore incorrect to classify preschoolers as totally "nonstrategic" but, like most components of development, strategy use develops gradually and has early precursors (DeLoache, 1985; Ornstein & Baker-Ward, 1983; Wellman, Fabricius, & Sophian, 1985; Wellman, Ritter, & Flavell, 1975). For example, when told what to buy at the store, a preschooler might repeat the words or look at the item longer than otherwise. The developmental fact that young children are capable of self-directed memory activity, but only in concrete practical activities, suggests that an early phase of strategy instruction in rehabilitation may be to encourage simple, concrete strategies in concrete activities before the child is at an age or point in recovery at which strategy acquisition can be addressed explicitly.

Assessment of Memory in Young Children

Given the complexity of memory and the many aspects of cognitive functioning that influence a child's ability to learn and remember, assessment is understood more properly as an exploration of relevant variables, including both standardized and informal procedures, than as the administration of memory tests alone. This is particularly true if the goal of assessment is to plan rehabilitation, and not just to establish levels of performance. Because setting appropriate expectations, determining treatment goals and procedures, and defining the best methods of instruction hang in the balance, this exploration should be undertaken with great care.

Preschoolers are particularly difficult to assess, because their performance is often more a function of their interest in the task than their ability to perform it. Furthermore, there are few normative data for the tasks listed below. Therefore, the point of this assessment is not primarily to establish the presence or absence of deficits; rather, it is to gain a useful description of the child's functioning in order to plan treatment and prescribe instructional methods.

The assessment tasks that follow are derived largely from memory research paradigms. The tasks are useful in probing the functioning of preschool children as well as older individuals in the early to middle stages of cognitive recovery from traumatic brain injury. Used cautiously, these tasks may serve as models for the development of treatment procedures for these groups, in that the tasks are consistent with the young child's capabilities and orientation. The research paradigms are discussed by Schneider and Pressley (1989), Flavell (1985), Siegler (1986), and Kail (1984).

Memory assessment is particularly important for children following traumatic brain injury because of the pervasiveness of memory and new learning problems. Tasks relevant to young or very impaired children are useful in planning early intervention and possibly even "preventive" therapy in the case of preschoolers. Tasks that address strategic behavior help clinicians structure their promotion of a "strategic attitude" early in the school years, thereby helping children with limited processing resources during their critical early learning years.

In interpreting these tasks, one must be sensitive to the distinctions between *encoding* (i.e., acquisition of information, construction of an internal representation of a perceived event), *storage* (i.e., holding information over time in an organized long-term memory system), and *retrieval* (i.e., transfer of information from long-term memory to consciousness). Retrieval is called *recognition memory* when the stimulus is present and one only needs to identify it (e.g., identifying objects as having been seen before, yes/no questions), *cued recall* when cues are given to prompt retrieval (e.g., wh– questions), and *free recall* when the stimulus is not present and must be retrieved without cues (e.g., retelling a story with no picture or question cues). In normal development there is evidence of recognition memory early in infancy and cued recall at least within the second half of the first year (Kail, 1984).

Habituation Paradigm (Fagan, 1973)

The infant is presented with a series of recurring patterns on a screen followed by a novel pattern. Special attention to the new pattern suggests recognition of the old pattern and therefore of the novelty of the new pattern. Recognition memory for visual patterns has been demonstrated in infants between 1 and 6 months. Procedures of this sort can be used to assess recognition in minimally responsive patients.

Conjugate Reinforcement Procedure (Rovee-Collier, 1984)

An interesting stimulus (e.g., mobile) is placed within view of the infant and is connected to a body part (e.g., ankle) by a ribbon so that the infant's movement will initiate activity in the stimulus. If the infant's movement increases (i.e., to make the event happen), the ribbon is detached and later reattached to determine if the rate of movement is greater than the original baseline. A higher rate of movement is evidence of recognition memory. Two-month-old infants have evidenced recognition memory using this procedure, with length of retention time steadily increasing over infancy. When adapted switches are connected to interesting electronically controlled events, this procedure can be used to assess recognition memory in minimally responsive head injury patients.

Memory for Location of Objects

Several types of tasks have been used to assess memory for location of objects. One simple procedure is to note all occurrences of the child looking for a misplaced object, or looking in the normal location for a desired object. Over the second half of the first year of life children evidence recall of fixed objects first (e.g., toybox), followed by movable objects (e.g., toys) (Ashmead & Perlmutter, 1980).

A second task is called hide-and-seek (DeLoache, Cassidy, & Brown, 1985). Here, one hides a desirable toy under a pillow and then plays with another attractive toy. The child's behavior is observed. Children at 18 to 24 months may interrupt their play to look at or point to the location of the hidden object.

Another task is retrieval of hidden objects with cues (Gordon & Flavell, 1977; Ritter, Kaprove, Fitch, & Flavell, 1973). In this task, the examiner compares the child's search for a hidden object when there is a picture (i.e., a cue) on the outside of the container in which the object is hidden and when there is no cue. Three year olds have been shown to use obvious, visible cues in such tasks. With older head injured children who demonstrate no spontaneous strategy use, this task helps to assess their readiness for prompted external strategy use.

A final task in this category is self-initiated cuing for retrieval of objects (Ritter, 1978). The examiner places candy in one of six cups. Pens, paper clips, or gold stars should be available to serve as markers for the cup that holds the candy. With the child's eyes closed, the examiner changes the location of the cups and then asks the child to locate the candy. If the child does not spontaneously mark the cup in order to find the candy after relocation, the examiner should provide increasingly explicit prompts, like "Is there something you can do to help yourself?" or "Can you use these stars to help find the candy?" Three year olds either fail to use the markers or require very concrete cuing. Five year olds need less cuing, and third graders use markers spontaneously. This is also a useful task for assessing strategy readiness in head injured children.

Memory for Events and Event Sequences

The examiner acts out a common script (i.e., an organized sequence of events) and asks the child to reconstruct the sequence. Or the examiner shows the child how to operate an interesting toy and probes recall after an interval. Two year olds are able to remember an interesting event for a short time. Memory is enhanced in preschoolers when the script is interesting. Preschoolers benefit from scripts in memory tasks, although their scripts may be general (Lucariello & Nelson, 1985).

Sort–Recall

Here the examiner helps the child to sort objects using different schemes and determines which is most useful in improving recall. Examiner-generated organization has been found to yield better recall in preschoolers than self-generated organization (Ceci, 1980). Prompted semantic sorting (e.g., into categories) improved the memory of 4 to 5 year olds. Nonprompted sorting of objects to enhance recall has not been observed in preschoolers. Observing which type of sorting helps recall most is useful in determining how the child organizes experience and therefore what type of information organization will help that child learn more efficiently. The child's performance in sort-and-remember tasks can be compared with play-and-remember tasks (Sodian, Schneider, & Perlmutter, 1986). Preschoolers' preference for thematic over categorical organization is discussed in the next section.

Deliberate Versus Involuntary Memory

Holding everything else constant, the examiner gives the child a memory task with and without the instruction to remember. As discussed earlier, preschoolers generally perform better when they are oriented only to the task itself and not to the need to remember (assuming an interesting and meaningful task). An individual who performs much better in involuntary memory tasks may not be a candidate for training in compensatory strategies or may require considerable attention to prerequisites for strategic behavior.

Listen/View Versus Play Versus Practical Activity

Holding other things constant, the examiner can compare memory performance when the objects to be remembered are (1) presented in the context of a practical activity (e.g., getting items needed to make a project), (2) presented in the context of play, or (3) simply named, viewed, and manipulated by the child. Preschoolers often perform best in the context of practical activity, least well if there is no play or practical activity associated with the task.

Teach New Material

Perhaps the most important component of memory/learning assessment in preschoolers (and older children) who appear to have recovered well after traumatic brain injury is to teach *new* information (e.g., vocabulary, rules, routines, routes, or games not known pretraumatically) under optimal as well as normal conditions for learning, and to observe the child's rate of learning and effectiveness of retention.

Various studies have revealed enormous variability in 5 year olds' memory, depending on features of the task (Istominia, 1977; Myers & Perlmutter, 1978; Perlmutter & Ricks, 1979; Szekeres, 1988). The mean number of items recalled has varied from three to seven. There is a general tendency for recall of categorically organized objects to be better than recall for unrelated objects, and recall for thematically related events to be even better.

These probes are designed to explore how effectively a given child learns or remembers under varying conditions. Understanding the best conditions for learning enables teachers and therapists to present new information and skills in a way that makes most efficient use of the child's memory system. In addition, decisions can more easily be made about the child's readiness for the next stage of memory development (e.g., learning to use memory strategies).

Normal Development of Conceptual Organization

Children with traumatic brain injury frequently evidence disorders of organizational functioning, which are demonstrated by disorganized activities of daily living, poorly organized expressive language (e.g., disjointed conversations and narratives), weak language comprehension because of difficulty integrating a text and seeing the main point, and weak retention of new information because it was not adequately integrated with existing knowledge at the time of encoding. Understanding how a child organizes experiences helps clinicians to present new information in a way that is easiest for the child to process and learn. It also helps to identify goals for organizational functioning, ultimately leading to the deliberate use of organizational strategies in learning and problem solving.

Organization can be thought of as a product, process, or conceptual structure (Pelligrino & Ingram, 1978). As a *product*, organization is the stable and identifiable relationship among organized items (Mandler, 1967). For example, when chairs are lined up theater style in a room, that is their organization. As a *process*, organizing is something that people do when they arrange objects, events, or ideas according to some principle. Organizing generally involves a goal, a plan based on a survey of the items or ideas, and manipulation of the items or ideas while monitoring and evaluating the product. Effective organizing of experience and behavior allows individuals to function efficiently in a complex environment and to deal with amounts of information that far exceed memory capacity.

Organization as a *conceptual structure* is the mental representation of organizational principles, which is hypothesized to explain an individual's organizing of objects, people, events, or ideas into a pattern. For example, when a child retells a story in a way that follows a pattern for story telling, it is assumed that he or she has that story schema as a guiding conceptual structure, a structure that may also enhance comprehension of stories.

Organizational Schemes

There are countless ways in which things, events, and ideas can be organized. Examples of common organizational schemes that figure prominently in the daily life and academic functioning of children include the following:

Perceptual Similarity. Arranging items according to color, shape, size, sound, texture, taste, and the like.

Semantic Relations. Arranging items according to features such as supraordinate categories (e.g., dogs and cats are animals), part–whole relations, or opposites.

Function (Use). Grouping items that share a function (e.g., brush, rag, soap, pail, and sponge go with washing a car).

Main Idea and Detail (Discourse Structure). Grouping related facts under the main idea that holds the facts together.

Story Schema. Grouping people and events in a story under headings like setting, characters, episodes, barriers, and solutions (Rummelhart, 1975).

General Life Scripts. Grouping biographical events under broad categories, such as time and place of birth, time and place of education, time and place of marriage and jobs.

Specific Event Scripts. Grouping things or events according to sequences that are common in life. For children, typical specific event scripts are getting up and getting ready for school, going to school, going to a birthday party, visiting the doctor, going camping, and many more (Bower & Black, 1979).

Assessment of Organization

A variety of research tasks have been used to gain insight into the semantic organization of preschool children. These include:

Sorting Tasks. The child puts objects, pictures, or words into groups and possibly also identifies the relation that exists among the items. The Word Association Subtest of the Word Test (Jorgenson, Barrett, Huisingh, & Zachman, 1981) is an illustration of this task standardized for grade school–age children.

Word Association Tasks. The child responds freely to a stimulus word. Based on this type of evidence, several investigators have identified an organizational shift from syntagmatic or functional associations (e.g., eat–cake, throw–ball) to paradigmatic associations (e.g., cake–pie, ball–glove) (Entwisle, 1966; Petrey, 1977). This shift is said to occur in the early grades, but there is evidence that all types of association can occur earlier. Developmentally earlier associations may tend to be more idiosyncratic (e.g., pie–Grandma or pie–sick), based on the preschoolers' tendency to organize things and ideas based on potent real-life experiences.

Word Definition. The examiner determines whether the child tends to define words in terms of function, category, synonym, strong association, or by some other mechanism.

Word Recognition. The child indicates words that were previously heard or seen. The examiner determines if there is a pattern to the words most readily recognized.

Sort–Recall Tasks. The child sorts objects into groups; this is followed by a recall test. It is important to determine which type of sorting promotes the best memory performance.

Observation of the Child's Spontaneous Organization in Play, Practical Activity, and Test Tasks. Here the examiner determines how effectively and in what ways the child spontaneously organizes things. It is important to use both intrinsically structured tasks (e.g., playing with representational toys, making a sandwich) and tasks without intrinsic structure (e.g., making something out of Tinker Toys).

Storytelling Tasks. Here the examiner asks the child to tell a story about some familiar character (e.g., G. I. Joe). The story's organization can be analyzed using story grammar categories (Hedberg & Westby, 1991; Stein & Glenn, 1979).

Descriptions. The examiner asks the child to describe familiar people, objects, or events. Organizational features of the description can be analyzed using developmental levels of narrative organization (Hedberg & Westby, 1991)

Organization and Memory

Memory research with all age groups has consistently demonstrated a close relationship between organization and memory. Well-organized information is learned more readily and remembered longer than poorly organized information (Bower, 1972). However, encoding, storage, and retrieval are facilitated only when the way in which the information is organized "fits the learner's head"; that is, it is congruent with the organizational structures available in the learner's semantic memory (Brown, 1975, 1979; Hagen, Jongeward, & Kail, 1975). This notion of "headfitting" is a useful concept in memory therapy and instructional design.

If organization of material is to help, then it has to appear organized to the child (Lange, 1978). Research in this area has focused on comparisons of the effects of perceptual, categorical, and thematic organization on memory. Although a preschooler's memory may be facilitated by any of these forms of organization, it appears that young children may prefer thematic organization, that is, the presentation of information in the context of real-life functional relationships, scripts, or stories (Ceci & Howe, 1978; Szekeres, 1988). Furthermore, preschoolers, unlike older children, profit from organization in the material to be learned when the organization of the material is imposed externally and highlighted verbally by the adult (Baumeister & Smith, 1979; Ceci, 1980; Horowitz, Lampel, & Takanishi, 1969; Moely, 1977); that is, young children are not *active* organizers in learning tasks.

Treatment Considerations: Organization and Memory in Young Children

The developmental findings noted previously have two primary implications for the treatment and education of young children following brain injury or older children with significant cognitive impairment following brain injury: (1) learning of new information or skills will likely be enhanced if the information is presented in a specific manner (e.g., personally meaningful involuntary learning tasks) and within an organizational structure (e.g., familiar thematic organization) that "fits the child's head"; and (2) cognitive recovery or development may be promoted by teaching the child new organizational schemes. Treating memory as an autonomous "muscle" to be exercised in a "muscle-building" manner has been found ineffective in the treatment of brain injured adults (Moffat, 1984; Schacter & Glisky, 1986) and children with other disabilities (Belmont & Butterfield, 1971).

Several features have been identified as useful in designing treatment programs. These are discussed next.

Task Design

In general, preschoolers learn most efficiently when they are engaged in tasks that are interesting and personally meaningful, that have a concrete goal rather than the abstract goal of learning something, and that have the target information *highlighted* and *organized* with other information in a way that is meaningful for that child.

Acquisition of Organized Knowledge

Because a rich and well-organized knowledge base improves processing of new information, building content knowledge and building associations among the elements in semantic memory are a part of "memory rehabilitation," understood very broadly. This includes facilitating the acquisition or reacquisition of meaningful scripts through dramatic play (e.g., getting up and getting ready for school, going to the doctor, going camping) and elaborating upon old ideas by identifying new features and relations. These scripts may have to be rehearsed many times and perhaps written by the child and clinician so that they also can be reviewed with the child by parents. Later, clinicians can promote the use of these associations in recall tasks. For example, in writing a story for mom about a visit to the doctor, the practiced script is used to make sure that all of the relevant events are mentioned. In this way, the child uses—with coaching—the types of organization-based memory strategies that may later be used internally. Table 6.1 lists a variety of activities designed to improve the organizational functioning and understanding of adolescents. When developmentally appropriate tasks are included, the same types of activities are useful with younger children.

Early Strategic Behavior

Given that the movement from involuntary to deliberate learning behavior and from externally to internally initiated strategic behavior is along a continuum (Flavell, 1986), clinicians working with older preschoolers and children moving out of the confused stages of recovery should begin to elicit concrete strategic behavior in the context of high-interest play or practical activity (e.g., marking the cup in which the candy is stored). External cues such as markers on boxes to indicate their content, a schedule card to remain oriented, and posted task reminders to stay on task are useful precursors to later strategy use.

Metamemory

Although normally developing preschoolers are not expected to have anything more than a rudimentary understanding of their own memory,

Table 6.1. Reestablishing organized semantic memory.

Organizational schema (means for attaining the goal)	Task and goal	Activity	Reflection[a]
Perceptual similarity (e.g., color, shape, size, texture, rhyme)	"The shop asked us to organize these leftover pieces of sandpaper so they can easily be found. Let's find a good way to do this."	Label small boxes for different grains (extra fine, fine, medium, etc.). Sort the pieces according to their "texture" and put them into the labeled boxes. Call out the textures and time how quickly they can be found.	How did you sort? Why this way? Was it "good"? In what other situations might one sort by texture? What would have happened if you had sorted by size? How could this help you remember where your tools or other possessions are kept or at least help you always locate them?
Semantic similarity (e.g., superordinate category, opposites)	"We got a job to set up the layout of a new department store. We have to make it easy for customers to find what they want."	Make a floor plan specifying the location of departments. Place labeled items into the departments, grouping them by similarity (e.g., TVs, stereos, radios) in one area, but sub-grouped within the area. Make display arrangement to entice people to buy (e.g., comfortable chair, flowers, glass of wine, and stereo).	How did you arrange the store? Why did you use that arrangement? In what other situations would you group things this way? When would this arrangement be inconvenient? How could knowing this arrangement help your memory of a visit to a store? How did the display arrangement differ from the floor arrangement?
Function (use)	"We are moving furniture into a new house. We have to arrange the living room for TV watching and conversation."	Make a floor plan and arrange labeled blocks representing the furniture. Then rearrange them for special occasions, such as a cocktail party or a Tupperware party.	How were the items arranged for each activity? Why did you have to change them? How is this different from a department store arrangement?

continued

Table 6.1. *Continued*

Organizational schema (means for attaining the goal)	Task and goal	Activity	Reflection[a]
Main idea and topic (discourse structure)	"We will present today's news to the orientation group." (Watch a videotaped news item or listen to an audiotaped news item.)	Listen to the tape. Fill in a form answering Who, What, When, Where, Why, and What happened questions and identifying the main idea. Relate the news item to another person using the diagram as notes.	How did the form help you remember? When wouldn't the form help? How did you stay so organized and coherent when you related the news item?
Story schema (Rummelhart, 1975)	"We will share a short story or TV show with those unable to see or hear it".	Watch the videotape of a TV show or listen to an audiotape of a radio show. Fill out a schema diagram, including characters, setting, and episodes. Retell the story using the organizational diagram as a cue.	How did this form help you remember? How is the information arranged? Why is this arrangement good for a story? Would it be good for a math book? Why not?
General life scripts (abstracted common life events)	"We will write our autobiographies and present a 'this is your life' program."	Fill out a form with labeled boxes of common life events (birth, school, marriage, job) and uncommon significant events (e.g., head injury). Using the form as a guide, write the autobiography and then present it formally in a radio program format.	How did the form make writing more organized? How could the form help reconstruct the past? How is your autobiorgaphy organized (e.g., chronologically)? How did the written preparation help the oral presentation?
Specific event scripts (e.g., going to a restaurant, going to the dentist)	"We will explain to [*a small child*] what it will be like when he has to go to the dentist.	Fill in a form with relevant information about the situation to prepare what you are going to say to the child:	How did this form help you? Why wouldn't a general life script help you? How is your explanation to the child organized?

Table 6.1. *Continued*

Organizational schema (means for attaining the goal)	Task and goal	Activity	Reflection[a]
		Who will be there: Equipment. Sequence of expected events and actions. Expected layout of the room and some variations. Then using the guide, explain to a child or explain in a role-playing situation.	Why would this help you remember what has happened to you?

[a] Possible probe questions to develop metacognition, understanding, and awareness.
Note. From "Topics in Cognitive Rehabilitation Therapy" (p. 165–168) by M. Ylvisaker, S. Szekeres, K. Henry, D. M. Sullivan, and P. Wheeler, in *Community Re-entry for Head Injured Adults* edited by M. Ylvisaker and E. M. R. Grobble, 1987, San Diego: College-Hill Press. Copyright 1987 by College-Hill Press/Little, Brown. Reprinted with permission.

promoting this awareness may be useful for children with cognitive impairment, due to the intimate relationship between metamemory and the acquisition of memory strategies. Words like "remember," "forget," "guess," and "know" can be highlighted in meaningful activity. Children can practice predicting their performance in tasks, including memory tasks, as a means to acquiring a greater awareness of memory.

Efficiency

The efficiency with which information is processed is, in part, a function of the automaticity of components of the task. Associations and skills become automatic through practice. Therefore, overlearning of information and skills is critical for young children and children with significant cognitive impairment.

Teaching Compensatory Cognitive Strategies

The domain of cognitive rehabilitation for school-age children and adolescents whose recovery is beyond the stage of significant confusion includes (1) identification of the conditions under which the child learns and performs most effectively, and manipulation of the environment and instructional practices to maximize performance; (2) instruction in academic content and general knowledge, including concepts and their organization, on the assumption that an enriched knowledge base enhances efficiency of information processing; (3) practice in specific cognitive processes (e.g., perceptual processes, problem-solving processes) if the processes lend themselves to practice effects (which may not be the case with general cognitive functions like memory); (4) teaching of compensatory strategies; and (5) intervention designed to heighten metacognitive awareness and executive control over cognitive behavior. The first two categories relate primarily to the goal of enhancing the *products* of learning, that is, increasing the student's body of knowledge and skill. The remaining categories, on the other hand, are *process* goals designed to help students improve the way they learn and solve problems. The latter has been a primary focus of educational theory and practice in recent years (Weinstein & Mayer, 1986).

Teaching a child to learn more efficiently by deliberately using complex study procedures, or by using a complex internal manipulation of information to make it more memorable, has a variety of developmental prerequisites. Therefore, this mode of intervention is inappropriate for young children or children who, following brain injury, are in the stage of recovery characterized by disorientation and shallow, egocentric thinking. However, because both normal cognitive development and typical recovery from brain injury proceed along a complex set of continua, and because individual strategies vary in their prerequisites, it would be misguided to seek clear criteria separating strategic children from nonstrategic children and to restrict strategy intervention to those children who meet these criteria. Promoting strategic behavior begins with the simple, concrete, externally focused strategic activities mentioned in the previous section, which can be relevant to children at a 4 to 5 year level of functioning. At the other extreme are elaborate study procedures relevant to college students whose recovery may be nearly complete.

Cognitive strategies—procedures used to enhance performance on cognitively demanding tasks—may involve the use of external aids (e.g., written reminder, printed schedule, memory book, printed task organizer), overt behavior (e.g., asking for information to be repeated, counting on fingers, repeating information out loud), or covert behavior (e.g., mentally rehearsing, elaborating, or organizing information; guiding oneself through a task with covert instructions). In normal development and also in recovery from brain injury, strategic behavior progresses from externally prompted use of simple external aids to internally prompted use of more elaborate internal procedures. Although the term "strategy" often is applied to the teachers' or clinicians' instructional procedures, we restrict this discussion to those procedures that the child uses to improve performance.

Three decades of accumulated research have shown that children in the early grades and children with mild to moderate cognitive impairment profit from experimenter-prompted mnemonic strategies. However, only older and cognitively more intact children evidence transfer of strategic behavior to similar tasks, maintenance of the behavior over time, and effective use of strategic procedures without prompting (Brown & Barclay, 1976; Butterfield & Belmont, 1977; Keeney, Cannizzo, & Flavell, 1967; Pressley & Levin, 1983a, 1983b). These findings motivated research in metacognitive development and its relation to the acquisition of functional strategic behavior. They also forced researchers and clinicians to be more thoughtful in the selection of candidates for strategy intervention, in the selection of specific strategies, and in the selection of teaching procedures, particularly focusing on generalization and maintenance.

Selecting Candidates for Strategy Intervention: Assessment

The growing literature on procedures for teaching cognitive strategies (Alley & Deshler, 1979; Brown, 1974; Deshler, Alley, Warner, & Schumaker, 1981; Forrest-Pressley, MacKinnon, & Waller, 1985a,b; Meichenbaum, 1977; Pressley & Levin, 1983a) unfortunately has not been paralleled by the development of techniques for assessing children's functioning in areas related to strategy use. Consequently, there are no simple measures or clear indicators available to determine if a child is a good candidate for this type of intervention.

Knowing the characteristics of mature, effective strategy users helps clinicians identify the areas that require careful assessment and also suggests broad goals for this type of intervention. The following list of attributes of good strategy users is modified from the model presented by Pressley, Goodchild, Fleet, Zajchowski, and Evans (1989). Generally, assessment of children should include probes in each of the areas outlined by the attributes. At one extreme, children who already possess all of the attributes of good strategy users are not candidates for intervention because they are already adequately strategic. At the other extreme, children with substantial deficits in most or all of the areas may not be candidates until certain prerequisites are addressed. However, all of these areas could be legitimate targets for intervention as part of a total package of strategy training. The following have been identified as characteristics of good strategy users.

Good strategy users have *goals* to which strategies are relevant. This is especially germane for individuals with head injury. An organically based unawareness of deficit often combines with psychoreactive denial to create a situation in which children or adolescents do not recognize that they have problems and consequently lack an appreciation of the fact that they have goals that cannot be attained without the use of strategic procedures.

Good strategy users know *why* to use strategies. A component of metacognitive knowledge that supports strategy use is knowing that performance needs to be enhanced and that strategies will enhance performance, that is, enable one to meet one's goals more effectively. This knowledge applies both to specific strategic procedures (i.e., "specific strategy knowledge"; Borkowski, Weyhing, & Turner, 1986) and to general strategic activity (i.e., "general strategy knowledge").

Having children predict their performance on tasks and evaluate their performance after completion helps to determine their awareness of deficits and their capacity for performance monitoring. Individuals who are always confident that they will perform well or, alternatively, who believe that they will perform poorly and that superior performance is a matter of luck or raw ability rather than strategic effort will not be as receptive to strategy intervention as individuals who recognize that they need help and that there are things that they can do to improve their performance.

Good strategy users know that they are *capable* of using strategies. Interviewing children about what they do to help themselves perform difficult tasks—particularly cognitive or academic tasks—helps determine whether they have a general sense for strategic procedures and an understanding of the active role that they can play in learning or other demanding tasks. This interview may be conducted in the context of playing a complex game with the child.

Good strategy users know *when* and *where* to use strategies. One of the failures of early strategy intervention for intellectually impaired children was that the children were taught strategies as rote behaviors, despite the fact that many strategies are limited in their applicability. Simple rehearsal of words, for example, is useful in improving recall of word lists but is counterproductive if the goal is to understand and remember a lecture or conversation. Peer teaching exercises—having a child prescribe strategic behavior that would be helpful for a peer—is useful in revealing the child's understanding of when and where to use strategies. Strategy intervention must target this type of metacognitive knowledge, and training must include varied tasks, settings, and strategies so that the child's situational discrimination increases along with the use of strategies.

Good strategy users can *monitor* the effectiveness of performance, including strategic performance. Children who fail to monitor their performance are unlikely to acquire or maintain strategies. Because the use of strategies requires effort, it is necessary to receive feedback regarding their value in relation to meaningful goals. Asking children *how* and *how well* they performed a difficult task, particularly if they had been asked to use a strategy in performing the task, yields insight into the child's ability to monitor performance. Training that includes frequent, immediate, and clear feedback, preferably charted by the children themselves, is an important ingredient of strategy training. Initially, most children need teacher cues to monitor their use of strategies.

Good strategy users know *many strategies* and can *modify or combine* them as needed. Some strategies (e.g., first letter mnemonics) are limited to a very restricted domain of learning tasks. Others (e.g., checking one's work, paying careful attention to directions) are more generally applicable. Still others (e.g., summarizing or elaborating information in a text while studying for an exam) fall between these two extremes. Assessment of children's spontaneous use of strategies should occur in formal learning tasks and also in games, recreational reading, and practical activities (e.g., shopping). In each setting, children can be given tasks that are slightly beyond their capacity and thereby designed to elicit strategic behavior. Young children can be given highly motivating concrete problem-solving tasks designed to elicit concrete strategic procedures (e.g., getting candy out of a tightly closed container, getting cookies from a high shelf). The clinician should note all strategies used and their relevance and effectiveness.

Good strategy users can use strategies *automatically*. Although cognitive strategies begin as deliberate attempts to solve problems that are based on cognitive weakness, it is important to practice their use to the point of habituation. If strategic procedures do not become automatic, it is likely that they will be discarded because they require more effort than they are worth.

Good strategy users have adequate *attentional space* (i.e., working memory). If an older child or adolescent is able to repeat no more than three or four digits, it may be difficult for that child to hold a strategic thought in mind and also have adequate cognitive resources left to consider the task at hand. It is not clear that attentional space or short-term memory is "expandable" with memory drills. In this case, ensuring automaticity of strategic behavior would be mandatory. Alternatively, environmental cues and teacher-cued or initiated strategies may be the only alternatives.

Good strategy users are not overly *impulsive* or *anxious*. Extremely impulsive children may learn a strategy but not use it functionally because their impulsiveness leads them to act before taking critical information into account (Messer, 1976). Extremely anxious children exhaust limited cognitive resources on fear of failure or negative thoughts about themselves and therefore fail to execute the planning and problem solving that are associated with the use of strategies.

Good strategy users receive *support* from others in the environment for the use of strategies. Many strategies are potentially stigmatizing (e.g., requesting repetition or clarification of what was said, asking for more time to complete a task) or place a demand on parents or teachers (e.g., asking for instructions to be written in a special instruction book). Some parents and teachers mistakenly believe that strategies interfere with development or reacquisition of cognitive skills, or that their use is a sign of laziness. If parents and teachers fail to appreciate the need for strategies, they may discourage their use. Therefore, assessment of the attitudes of significant people in the environment is an important component of this intervention.

Good strategy users have an adequate fund of general *knowledge* to support the use of strategies. It is unlikely, for example, that a child who is asked to summarize a text about a completely unfamiliar topic will be able to make effective use of a text-organizing strategy. Certain strategies, particularly organizational strategies, presuppose a body of knowledge. *Content knowledge* can be assessed in a variety of familiar ways (e.g., achievement tests).

In addition, strategy use presupposes adequate general intellectual functioning and, in the case of brain injury, recovery beyond the stage of significant confusion. However, because strategy use as well as intellectual functioning and cognitive recovery occur in degrees, there are no clear cutoff points for the beginning of strategy exploration. Often the determination of a child's appropriateness for strategy intervention can be made only through a period of trial strategy teaching.

In summary, good strategy users are people who perform difficult tasks effectively because they are clever about finding alternative ways to perform the task. This implies (1) an understanding of their own ability, (2) an understanding of task demands, (3) an understanding of and facility with strategic procedures, (4) motivation to achieve the goal, and (5) support for strategic behavior.

Selecting Strategies

There is an important irony in the common clinical and educational practice of identifying a child's deficit (e.g., inefficient comprehension of extended text), selecting a strategy that is designed to compensate for the deficit (e.g., a summarizing/note-taking strategy using wh–questions), and training the child to use the strategy. Strategic behavior is, essentially, active, problem-solving behavior. If the child lacks an appreciation of the problem, lacks motivation to perform better, does not see the point of the strategy, or finds the strategy objectionable in some way, then there is little chance that this instructional practice will succeed. The extent to which even impaired learners are capable of actively creating strategies to compensate for cognitive or academic weakness is easily underestimated (Belmont & Butterfield, 1971; Belmont, Ferretti, & Mitchell, 1982; Brown, 1974). Therefore, although there are criteria useful in the selection of strategies, it is critical to consider the selection of strategies as a process of *negotiation* between student and teacher/clinician. The process often begins with tasks designed to reveal the need for improved performance in areas clearly related to the student's goals, followed by brainstorming on procedures that may promote improved performance. The following factors should be considered seriously in selecting strategies.

Spontaneous Use

Other things being equal, the procedures that a student uses spontaneously have a distinct advantage over procedures that are new. For example, if during word-list learning tests the student is observed to associate by meaning or to create visual images, then these procedures should be made explicit and explored as potentially useful strategies in comprehending and remembering text. Alternatively, if the student asks for repetition or attempts to take notes, then the usefulness of these procedures should be explored in practical tasks.

Following brain injury, however, strategies that were successful before may now be ineffective. For example, a student who successfully prepared for a test by highlighting the main ideas in the text and reviewing these highlighted items, may be unable to identify the main ideas after the injury. There may be tension between the student's strategic inclinations and the professional judgment of the clinician, which again is best resolved by means of open negotiation and systematic exploration of the relative effectiveness of alternative procedures.

Difficulty of Use

Some procedures are difficult and time consuming. The well-known SQ3R method (i.e., Survey, Question, Read, Recite, Review) for studying text, for example, is so demanding that it could reasonably be expected to be used only if the payoffs were very large. Others are quite simple. Because difficulty is related to individual strengths and weaknesses, this variable is also subject to individual negotiation. For example, apparently simple procedures like asking for help or taking simple notes may be very difficult for students who have impaired initiation or who are emotionally unable to reveal their disability.

Concreteness

Other things being equal, students who are young or significantly impaired can learn to use and benefit from concrete external procedures (e.g., using an assignment book, following a printed or pictured task guide), but they may struggle with more abstract internal procedures (e.g., mentally elaborating information to make it more memorable). Concrete thinking is a common characteristic of individuals with traumatic brain injury.

Domain of Applicability

For some individuals, there are advantages in strategic procedures that apply only to the setting and task in question. For example, an impaired adolescent may be able to learn and benefit from a strategy for organizing and sequencing specific vocational tasks in a sheltered workshop setting. Transfer to other tasks and generalization to other settings may be unrealistic goals. In other cases, strategies that are broadly applicable (e.g., checking work, asking for clarification, writing important information in a memory book) may be preferable, if the student is capable of generalization, because training in generalizable strategies has greater cognitive and academic payoff. It is unfortunate that much of the research on the effectiveness of training in memory strategies has involved strategies with limited practical application (e.g., verbal rehearsal or mnemonic "tricks" like first letter acronyms) (Wilson & Moffat, 1984).

Neuropsychological Strengths

Clearly, students should be guided to select strategies that capitalize on their strengths. Students with a language impairment, for example, should avoid verbal elaboration as a procedure for improving text comprehension and memory. Students who are very shy are unlikely to maintain a strategy of requesting help. Students with visual-spatial orientation problems may be confused by organizational guides that take the form of printed diagrams or flow charts.

In summary, due to the importance of active student participation and to the complexity of the issues, selection of strategies is most usefully understood as a process of negotiation and systematic exploration of procedures that may help students do something that they want to do. The Appendix lists a variety of procedures that may be useful in promoting improved performance of academic or other cognitively demanding tasks. Weinstein and Mayer (1986) present an alternative scheme for categorizing strategies and a number of examples of strategies in each category.

Teaching Procedures

Many of the principles and techniques relevant to teaching compensatory strategies to brain injured students apply equally to the teaching of any skill. These include (1) careful task analysis; (2) systematic progression from simple, easy-to-master components to more complex procedures; (3) gradual fading of cues and prompts that were designed specifically at each stage to ensure success; (4) limited goals, so the student can see the task as manageable and complete it successfully; (5) reasonable criterion levels, again based on what the student can reasonably be expected to master; and (6) some fun in the process.

The acquisition phase of strategy instruction begins with a description of the strategic procedure, including both what the student is expected to do and what purpose the strategy is supposed to serve. Teacher or peer modeling, with elicited imitation, adds a needed concrete element to the verbal description so that the behavior expected of the student is amply clear. During the modeling, effective teachers include planned thinking out loud to ensure that the student understands not only the specific overt behavior but also the cognitive processes underlying the behavior and the purpose(s) that this behavior serves. The student should be encouraged to ask questions during the modeling and then to rehearse the strategy.

Given the cognitive and psychosocial characteristics of many students with head injury, additional techniques are designed specifically to capture and retain student engagement in the process and to ensure that strategies are not simply rote behaviors or isolated academic skills. Some of these are discussed next.

"Product-Monitoring" Tasks

On these tasks, the student is asked to perform a meaningful activity with and without the strategic procedure and then to evaluate the "products," that is, how well he or she performed the task under the two conditions. This focus on self-evaluation should continue throughout the training.

Explicit Feedback on Utility

This is the "sales pitch" that an effective teacher or clinician uses to promote a strategy that may be difficult or embarrassing. This includes brainstorming about varied uses of the strategy in varied settings.

Ongoing Negotiation/Modification

Students should be invited to consider modifying the strategies that they use based on their success or on other considerations. For example, a student may wish to give up a large memory book in exchange for a more discrete memo pad; a student who no longer feels that it is necessary to take elaborate notes may propose simply highlighting important points in the text.

Transferring Control from Teacher to Student

An important goal of strategy training is to increase independence. This requires that the teacher turn over the regulatory aspect of strategic behavior to the student. The alternative is to invite learned helplessness, a characteristic seen in many children with mental retardation.

Techniques for Overcoming Resistance

These include counseling and promotional techniques that focus on the *affective* component of strategy use. Images and metaphors are often useful (e.g., "This is like Joe Montana wearing a back brace when he was hurt"), as are testimonials from trusted peers.

Generalization and Maintenance

Finally, there are techniques designed to enhance generalization of the strategic behavior from task to task and setting to setting and help maintain the strategy over time. These include (1) training in the context of actual academic materials and activities, and systematically varying person, place, time, and activity once the strategy is initially acquired; (2) extensive practice to promote habituation and automatization; (3) gradual fading of teacher prompts; and (4) specific training in discriminating situations that call for the strategy. Care must be taken to ensure that all of the student's teachers understand the strategy and support its use.

An alternative solution to the generalization problem is to give up the goal of generalization. Students are simply trained to use a specific procedure for a specific task in a specific context. Ongoing use of the strategy is ensured by means of cue cards or teacher/supervisor prompts. This solution is particularly relevant for those students with substantial cognitive limitations and a degree of concreteness that makes flexible generalization of skills an unrealistic goal. Prevocational students, for example, may improve performance with a task-organizing strategy for a specific task in a specific work setting without being expected to transfer this skill to other tasks.

Efficacy Research

There exist no reports in the research literature on the effectiveness of strategy intervention with children and adolescents with traumatic brain injury. Although many clinicians have considered traumatic brain injury a disability category, and have explored this type of intervention with the population (Haarbauer-Krupa, Henry, Szekeres, & Ylvisaker, 1985), the relevant empirical data base exists in research with students with learning disabilities or mental retardation. Because these children may have different characteristics from children with traumatic brain injury, care must be exercised in generalizing positive or negative efficacy reports to this disability group.

However, the large body of literature that deals with other special education groups is very useful in highlighting critical aspects of the intervention (e.g., student involvement, systematic and intensive training, generalization and maintenance) and in supporting a cautious optimism that strategy training can be useful for well-selected students. As Meichenbaum and Asarnow (1979) observed, when strategy instruction is successful, it is hard to know whether the improvement is a result of improved problem solving in general, acquisition of a task-specific strategy, explicit feedback, the child's active engagement in the process, individually tailored instruction, or some other factor.

Approaches have included strategies curricula for specific academic skills (e.g., Alley & Deshler, 1979; Deshler, Alley, Warner, & Schumaker, 1981) as well as programs for improving strategic behavior in relation to more general aspects of cognitive or social functioning (e.g., Feuerstein, 1979, 1980; Meichenbaum, 1977). Recent summary textbooks that are worth review include Pressley and Brainerd (1985), Pressley and Levin (1983a, 1983b), and Forrest-Pressley, MacKinnon, and Waller (1985a, 1985b). Table 6.2 lists selected studies that support strategy intervention in relation to varied cognitive and academic goals.

Executive Functions and Cognitive Rehabilitation

Applied metacognitive research since the mid-1970s has been motivated in large part by the failure of early attempts to teach strategies to students with cognitive impairment (Brown, 1981; Flavell, 1976; Meichenbaum & Asarnow, 1979; Wong, 1986). When strategic procedures were taught as specific skills, they typically lacked durability and did not generalize to other tasks or settings (Borkowski & Cavanaugh, 1979; Campione & Brown, 1977; Keeney et al., 1967). An explanatory hypothesis for this phenomenon that gained wide acceptance was that the children lacked an awareness of the problem that the strategy was designed to solve (i.e., their deficient performance), an appreciation of the relation between their deficit and their goals, recognition of the characteristics of the tasks that made them difficult, and an understanding of the strategy that facilitated their performance. Alternatively, the children may have had an intellectual understanding of their cognitive strengths and weaknesses and deficient performance, and an understanding that strategies improved performance (i.e., the *static* aspects of metacognition), but they simply failed to *use* the strategies without prompts (i.e., the *dynamic* or *self-regulatory* aspect of metacognition) (Ylvisaker & Szekeres, 1989). Coupled with the emphasis in recent cognitive theory on the mind as an active information processor and problem solver (Anderson, 1975), this hypothesis has led to an enthusiastic reception of a metacognitive perspective among many educators (Wittrock, 1978) and special educators (Butterfield & Belmont, 1977; Wong, 1986).

A similar emphasis has evolved in head injury rehabilitation for both adults (Ben Yishay & Prigatano, 1989; Crosson et al., 1989; Prigatano, 1986) and children (Ylvisaker & Szekeres, 1989). The additional impetus in head injury, particularly closed head injury, is the pathophysiological fact that among the most vulnerable parts of the brain are parts of the frontal lobes associated with "executive" functioning. The territory covered by this metaphor includes most of what is traditionally included under the heading "metacognition." The executive system includes functions "necessary for formulating goals, planning how to achieve them, and carrying out the plans effectively" (Lezak, 1982). These functions include realistic goal setting, based on an awareness of one's strengths and weaknesses, planning, self-directing and initiating, self-inhibiting, self-monitoring, self-evaluating, self-correcting, and flexible problem solving.

Table 6.2. Cognitive strategy research: Selected references.

Cognitive domain	Reference
Component processes	
Attention	Brown & Alford, 1984
	Douglas, Parry, Marton, & Garson, 1976
	Hallahan & Reeve, 1980
	Kendall & Finch, 1978, 1979
	Nelson, 1985
Perception	Kavale & Mattson, 1983
	Keogh & Margolis, 1976
Memory/learning	Brown, 1974
	Brown & Campione, 1977
	Glidden & Warner, 1985
	Kirby, Nettlebeck, & Western, 1982
	Sabatino, Miller, & Schmidt, 1981
	Taylor, 1982
Organization	Ashcraft & Kellas, 1974
	Pieper & Deshler, 1985
	Merrill, 1985
	Shields & Heron, 1989
Reasoning/problem solving	Alley & Deshler, 1979
	Ewing & Brecht, 1977
	Gogue & Smith, 1962
	Goldman & Goldman, 1974
	Levine & Langness, 1983
	McKinney & Haskins, 1980
	McKinney & Keen, 1976
	Montague & Bos, 1986
	Patton & Griffin, 1973
	Urbain & Kendall, 1980
Component systems	
Working memory	Cermak, Goldberg, Cermak, & Drake, 1980
	Torgesen, 1988
Executive system	Bos, 1988
	Cohen & deBettencourt, 1983
	Englert & Raphael, 1988
	Karoly, 1977, 1984
	Keller & Hallahan, 1987
	Kneedler & Hallahan, 1981
	Loper, 1980
	Nettlebeck & McLean, 1984
	Paris & Oka, 1986
	Pressley, 1979
	Rooney & Hallahan, 1988
	Seabaugh & Schumaker, 1981
Functional-integrative performance	
Social Skills	Flaro, 1987
	Gresham, 1981
Reading	Jamison & Shevitz, 1985
	Marzola, 1988
	Shapiro & McCurdy, 1989
	Torgesen, 1985, 1988
	Vellutino & Scanlon, 1986
Spelling	Cook, 1981
	Graham & Freeman, 1986
Writing	Bos, 1988
	Graham & Freeman, 1986
	Graham & Harris, 1988

In the later stages of recovery following head injury, it is common for the most debilitating deficits to include weak awareness of deficits (possibly combined with psychoreactive denial), unrealistic goal setting, poorly regulated initiation or inhibition of behavior, weak self-monitoring, and generally ineffective problem solving. Applied to academic and cognitive functioning, this means that students may fail (1) to use their cognitive skills effectively (e.g., failing to initiate a search of memory even if the information is present in long-term storage), (2) to monitor performance and hence to recognize the need to perform better or to use special procedures to enhance performance, (3) to appreciate the options that are open to them to improve performance, and (4) to generalize improvements from one task or setting to another. Recently, even mental retardation has come to be described in terms that emphasize self-regulatory impairment as opposed to weakness in specific intellectual processes or systems (Whitman, 1990).

There has been widespread agreement that adults with serious executive system impairments related to substantial frontal lobe damage are resolutely resistant to rehabilitative efforts (Lezak, 1987). For example, adults who simply do not initiate behavior are poor candidates for rehabilitation. Whether or not there is reason to be optimistic about improving children and adolescents with mild to moderate executive or metacognitive dysfunction awaits careful investigation. It is only recently that the components of executive functioning have been specifically targeted in carefully programmed training curricula (e.g., Meichenbaum, 1977; Van Reusen, 1987) and that educational and rehabilitative environments have been designed to promote executive or self-regulatory functioning throughout the day (Feuerstein, 1980; Ylvisaker & Szekeres, 1989).

Training the Components of Executive Functioning

Being "strategic" or being a good practical problem solver is a very complex skill. Thus training programs should begin by breaking this skill into manageable components and illustrating their meaning and importance in concrete terms. When these components are addressed within the context of challenging academic activities, it is difficult for students with cognitive impairment to grasp the specific "executive" target. The components of executive or self-regulatory functioning targeted for intervention may include self-appraisal of strengths and weaknesses, the ability to predict performance and set realistic goals, self-monitoring, self-evaluating, and problem solving. The training is most useful for adolescents with only mild to moderate cognitive weakness but potentially very significant deficits in executive functioning.

Van Reusen (1987) emphasized the importance of highlighting target executive skills in the context of enjoyable and nonchallenging tasks (e.g., throwing balls into a basket). It is critical that the task have clear and readily quantifiable criteria for success. The student is first asked to predict his or her own performance if given 10 shots. If performance is predicted without asking to try the task first, the clinician initiates discussion of the need for evidence of ability before predictions can be made or goals set. The student then practices the shot and makes a prediction (i.e., sets a goal).

The prediction is recorded and a meaningful reward is promised, contingent on the student's *performance matching the prediction*. This must be made very clear, because the first training goal is not excellent ball throwing but, rather, accurate self-appraisal and prediction of success. Performance is charted. Two or three times during the 10 shots the student is asked how he or she is doing and how performance compares to the original prediction. The student is also given the opportunity to do *something* that would facilitate winning the reward. The teacher or clinician should ensure that the student considers all of the possible options. For example, the student could *change the prediction*. If the student predicted 8 out of 10 successful shots and has only 3 out of the first 5, then he or she may have to lower the prediction (goal). This corresponds to the alteration of goals that may be necessary as students with head injury become increasingly aware of their limitations. The student also could *change the task*. The student should be encouraged to consider various ways in which the task could be changed. For example, the basket could be moved closer, a backboard cold be put behind it, or the basket or ball could be changed. These changes correspond to task or environmental modifications that may be necessary as part of a total package of compensation for cognitive deficits (e.g., fewer math problems on the page, shorter reading assignments, fewer distractions in the environment during work time, or large-print books). As a third option, the student could *change the way the task is done*. The student should be encouraged to think of alternative ways to perform the task, for example, by using an underhand as opposed to overhand throw or standing up while throwing. These changes correspond to compensatory strategies and this parallel should be made clear. Finally, *practice*. In this example, the student could be encouraged to ask for a few practice shots. This corresponds to the necessary component in acquiring any skill or substantial body of knowledge—practice and repetition.

In this manner, the student comes to understand the primary components of executive functioning and can deliberately practice their use. The exercise is designed to highlight self-appraisal (i.e., taking stock of how well one can perform a task), appropriate goal setting/predicting and adjustment, self-monitoring (i.e., paying attention to how well one is doing), self-evaluating (i.e., judging success of performance in relation to a goal), and problem solving (e.g., figuring out how to meet the goal regardless of how well one currently performs the task). It is also a useful context for mastering a metacognitive vocabulary (assuming that the clinician has chosen words that are meaningful for the student), for gaining facility in task analysis, and for attaining insight into the important role of compensatory strategies, task and environmental modifications, and practice.

It is often useful to find a metaphor or image that is more meaningful for adolescents than that of an "executive" and that helps trigger for the student all of the components of executive functioning. Given that many head injured students are active, sports-minded adolescents, the image of an internalized coach is well suited to this task. The student and teacher together may create a list of functions that the coach performs, and then discuss self-appraisal, goal setting, planning, self-directing, self-monitoring, self-evaluating, and problem solving (including strategic thinking) as roles of the internal self-coach comparable to the roles played by a team coach.

When these self-regulatory skills are solidly in place in concrete, non-threatening tasks, it is time to transfer them to more demanding cognitive or academic tasks. All of the components of the exercise can be present, for example, in math lessons where the prediction is the number of correctly solved problems or in reading comprehension exercises where the prediction is the number of questions correctly answered after the reading. Initially, the goal is not superior performance in math or reading; rather, it is improved self-appraisal of skill levels, active performance monitoring, accurate self-evaluation, and insightful and flexible brainstorming on how to improve performance—through practice, modifying the task, changing the way the task is done (i.e., strategies), or perhaps adjusting performance expectations to meet the realities of one's ability. These are the areas of functioning that the teacher should prompt, encourage, and reward.

As with all skills, executive or metacognitive (self-coaching) skills must be practiced in a variety of settings, in the context of a variety of tasks, with a variety of people, and with systematically decreasing cues to promote generalization and maintenance. Ideally, the educational environment, including teacher–student interaction, is designed to promote improved self-regulatory functioning throughout the instructional day.

Environmental Factors in the Development of Executive Functions

Meichenbaum and Asarnow (1979) called for an educational environment that is imbued with a concern for the process of learning and the cognitive autonomy of students. Promoting generalization of strategic behavior is perhaps best accomplished by creating an environment in which strategic thinking and metacognitive insight are pervasive features. In a school setting, such environments are characterized by a variety of teacher behaviors that go far beyond teaching specific curricular content. Similarly, in a home setting such an environment can be created through interaction between parents and children and by establishing a standing expectation for autonomous problem solving on the part of the child.

In classrooms sensitive to the need to promote increased autonomy and improved self-regulation in students, one expects to hear the following types of comments from teachers:

Good question! How do you suppose you could find the answer?
How do you think you'll do on your math? Why do you think that?
How are you doing on your math? Did you do as well as you thought you would do?
What was the hardest part of it for you? What made it hard?
How long did it take you to finish? Do you think you could cut that down by 5 minutes? How?
What is your goal in working on this assignment? How do you plan to achieve it?
What do you suppose you could do to get a higher grade? Good idea! Why don't you try it and let me know what happens? How did the strategy work?
Be sure to check your work before you hand it in.
Before you hand in your essay, read through it and indicate all of the problems you had with spelling, grammar, and organization. I'll give you extra credit if you can find your own errors.
I want you all to pair up, find out how well your partner understands the social studies lesson, and figure out some way to ensure that your partner does well on the test.
Has anybody found a good way to prepare for social studies tests? Is there anybody you know who is good at this kind of thing who might give you some tricks to make it easier—maybe you could find out how they take notes.
What helps you learn and remember new things? Lots of repetition? Saying it out loud? Making diagrams? Outlining? Teaching somebody else?

Reciprocal teaching, developed by Brown and Palinscar (Palinscar, 1986), includes a focus on reading comprehension strategies as well as a dialogue between teacher and student that incorporates these metacognitive or executive themes in daily interaction.

Individual Educational Plans (IEP's) tend to be dominated by specific measurable objectives in areas of specific academic content; for example, "John will read paragraphs from his social studies text and answer yes/no and multiple choice questions with 90% accuracy" or "John will complete two-column subtraction problems with regrouping with 90% accuracy." Although it is certainly essential for students to master basic academic content, IEP's for students with learning and executive system problems after head injury should include additional objectives such as the following:

John will set goals for each social studies test; actual grade will match prediction 75% of the time; in cases in which performance falls below prediction, John will discuss the reason for the grade with his teacher; he will then list at least five things that he could do to improve performance and will negotiate a strategy for improving performance.

John will decide what he needs to do to achieve his goal for each major test, and he will give the plan to the teacher.

John will select a strategy he feels will help him prepare for tests; he will record the strategy and the frequency of its use in his log book; after completing the tests, he will record the effectiveness of the strategy and modify it if it was unsuccessful.

John will develop a system to keep track of daily assignments; he will monitor completion of daily assignments in his log book; if completion falls below 90%, John will identify the reason why he is not completing his assignments (e.g., didn't understand the assignment, didn't remember to take the books home, didn't have time, forgot to bring the work back to school) and will generate an appropriate solution.

Parents figure most prominently in the growth of strategic or problem-solving ability in preschoolers. Unfortunately, the natural maturation of these skills may be inhibited by the understandable inclination of parents to take over the problem-solving role of their newly disabled child and to protect the child from frustration. Time also comes to be a critical element in that basic care may be more time consuming than before the accident, thereby reducing time for problem-solving exploration. However, because children with handicaps are more reliant on strategic thinking and problem-solving skills than are children whose automatic behavior serves them adequately, these skills must figure prominently in the cognitive rehabilitation of young children and the training of their parents.

Training of parents involves the following components: (1) sensitizing them to the importance of cognitive maturation and independent problem solving; (2) teaching them to identify problem-solving situations in the lives of young children; (3) teaching them to explore alternative solutions with the child; (4) teaching them to encourage trial-and-error experimentation with possible solutions; (5) teaching them to give useful feedback that highlights the value of clever solutions and at the same time rewards the child for independent and creative thinking.

It might be useful to present contrasting videotaped models of parents acting for the child or telling the child what to do versus guiding the child through exploration of possible solutions. This is combined with sensitive discussion of reasons why children who are never expected to think creatively or solve their own problems are unlikely to develop this important skill. Useful problem situations include retrieving a toy from an inaccessible shelf, getting candy from a tightly closed jar, and resolving a conflict between siblings over which TV show to watch. Clinicians can help parents create lists of everyday problem-solving situations and possible solutions that could be safely explored. This type of training has been shown to have a positive influence on the behavior of parents of young children with handicaps (Thompson & Hixon, 1984).

Conclusions

The territory covered by the term "cognitive rehabilitation" is extremely broad and includes the intervention of many rehabilitation and special education professionals. Most children following traumatic brain injury return to school, with its attendant demands on cognitive and behavioral integrity. It is therefore critical to do what can be done to enable the child to succeed with the cognitive skills that remain after the injury. We have discussed three important and overlapping domains of cognitive rehabilitation: organization and memory, compensatory strategies, and metacognitive/executive skills. Deficits in these areas are common following traumatic brain injury and have pervasive implications. The approaches to rehabilitation that we recommend are grounded in a substantial body of knowledge regarding cognitive development, efficacy research that has been conducted with children whose needs are similar to those of head injured children, and a growing body of clinical experience with this population.

During the next decade, children with traumatic brain injury increasingly will be singled out for special attention in rehabilitation centers and schools. To ensure appropriate services for these children, creative assessment procedures must be combined with criteria for services that are consistent with what is known about this group. Furthermore, researchers, clinicians, and teachers must cooperate in the systematic investigation of variables that affect outcomes. In the case of young children, this requires very long-term outcome studies to determine the effectiveness of early "preventive" therapy. Since this type of intervention often includes both environmental engineering and metacognitive instruction, the relative effectiveness of different environments (e.g., regular education classroom with modifications and supports versus special education classroom) and of alternative approaches to metacognitive intervention needs to be investigated.

Finally, no discussion of traumatic brain injury in children is complete without a call for increased efforts in accident prevention. The only way to deal effectively with head injury is to prevent it. Every community in the country should have an active bicycle helmet campaign, focusing on children in the 5 to 10 year range. Active promotion of effective restraints and car seats and enforcement of strict drunk driving laws are also necessary to reduce the monumental personal loss and enormous societal costs that tragically have come to be accepted as part of modern life.

References

Alley, G. R., & Deshler, D. D. (1979). *Teaching the learning disabled adolescent strategies and methods*. Denver: Love Publishing Co.

Anderson, J. R. (1975). *Cognitive psychology and its implications*. San Francisco: Freeman.

Ashcraft, M. H., & Kellas, G. (1974). Organization in normal and retarded children: Temporal aspects of storage and retrieval. *Journal of Experimental Psychology*, *103*, 502–508.

Ashmead, D., & Perlmutter, M. (1980). Infant memory in everyday life. In M. Perlmutter (Ed.), *New directions for child development: Vol 10. Children's memory*. San Francisco: Jossey-Bass.

Baumeister, A., & Smith, S. (1979). Thematic elaboration and proximity in children's recall, organization, and long term retention of sectorial materials. *Journal of Child Psychology*, *28*, 231–248.

Belmont, J., & Butterfield, E. (1971). Learning strategies as determinants of memory deficiencies. *Cognitive Psychology*, *2*, 411–420.

Belmont, J., & Butterfield, E. (1977). The instructional approach to developmental cognitive research. In R. Kail & J. Hagen (Eds.), *Perspectives on the development of memory and cognition* (pp. 437–481). Hillsdale, NJ: Erlbaum.

Belmont, J., Ferretti, R. P., & Mitchell, D. (1982). Memorizing: A test of untrained mildly retarded children's problem solving. *American Journal of Mental Deficiency*, *87*, 197–210.

Ben Yishay, Y., & Prigatano, G. (1990). Cognitive remediation. In M. Rosenthal, E. R. Griffith, M. R. Bond, & J. D. Miller (Eds.), *Rehabilitation of the adult and child with traumatic brain injury* (2nd ed., pp. 393–409). Philadelphia: F.A. Davis Co.

Bjorklund, D. (1985). The role of conceptual knowledge in the development of organization in children's memory. In M. Pressley & C. Brainerd (Eds.), *Basic processes in memory development* (pp. 103–134). New York: Springer-Verlag.

Borkowski, J. G., & Cavanaugh, J. C. (1979). Maintenance and generalization of skills and strategies by the retarded. In N. R. Ellis (Ed.), *Handbook of mental deficiency: Psychological theory and research* (2nd ed., pp. 569–618). Hillsdale, NJ: Erlbaum.

Borkowski, J. G., Johnston, M. B., & Reid, M. K. (1986). Metacognition, motivation, and the transfer of control process. In S. J. Ceci (Ed.), *Handbook of cognitive, social, and neuropsychological aspects of learning disabilities*. (pp. 147–173). Hillsdale, NJ: Erlbaum.

Borkowski, J. G., Weyhing, R. S., & Turner, L. A. (1986). Attributional retraining and the teaching of strategies. *Exceptional Children*, *53*, 130–137.

Bos, C. S. (1988). Process-oriented writing with mildly handicapped students. *Exceptional Children*, *54*, 521–527.

Bower, G. (1972). A selective review of organizational factors in memory. In E. Tulving & W. Donaldson (Eds.), *Organization of memory* (pp. 93–137). New York: Academic Press.

Bower, G., & Black, J. (1979). Scripts in memory for texts. *Cognitive Psychology*, *11*, 177–220.

Brink, J. D., Garret, A. L., Hale, W. R., Woo-Sam, J., & Nickel, V. L. (1970). Recovery of motor and intellectual functions in children sustaining severe head injuries. *Developmental Medicine and Child Neurology*, *12*, 565–571.

Brown, A. L. (1974). The role of strategic behavior in retardate memory. In N. R. Ellis (Ed.), *International review of research in mental retardation*, (Vol. 7, pp. 55–111). New York: Academic Press.

Brown, A. L. (1975). The development of memory: Knowing, knowing about knowing, and knowing how to know. In H. W. Reese (Ed.), *Advances in child development and behavior*. (Vol. 10, pp. 103–152). New York: Academic Press.

Brown, A. L. (1978). Metacognitive development and reading. In R. J. Spiro, B. C. Bruce, & G. W. Brewer (Eds.), *Theoretical issues in reading comprehension* (pp. 77–165). Hillsdale, NJ: Erlbaum.

Brown, A. L. (1979). Theories of memory and problems of development, activity, growth, and knowledge. In F. I. M. Craik & L. Cermak (Eds.), *Levels of processing and memory* (pp. 225–258). Hillsdale, NJ: Erlbaum.

Brown, A. L. (1981). Learning to learn: On training students to learn from texts. *Educational Researcher*, *10*, 14–21.

Brown, A. L., & Barclay, C. R. (1976). The effects of training specific mnemonics on the metamnemonic efficiency of retarded children. *Child Development*, *47*, 71–80.

Brown, A. L., & Campione, J. C. (1977). Training strategic study time appointment in educable retarded children. *Intelligence*, *1*, 94–107.

Brown, A. L., & Palincsar, A. S. (1982). Inducing strategic learning from text by means of informed, self-control training. *Topics in Learning and Learning Disabilities*, *2*, 1–17.

Brown, G., Chadwick, O., Shaffer, D., Rutter, M., & Traub, M. (1981). A prospective study of children with head injuries: III. Psychiatric sequelae. *Psychological Medicine*, *11*, 63–78.

Brown, R. T., & Alford, M. (1984). Ameliorating attentional deficits and concomitant academic deficiencies in learning disabled children through cognitive training. *Journal of Learning Disabilities*, *17*, 20–26.

Butterfield, E., & Belmont, J. (1977). Assessing and improving the executive cognitive functions of mentally retarded people. In I. Bialer & M. Sternlicht (Eds.), *The psychology of mental retardation: Issues and approaches* (pp. 277–315). New York: Psychological Dimensions.

Butterfield, E. C., Wambold, C., & Belmont, J. M. (1973). On the theory and practice of improving short-term memory. *American Journal of Mental Deficiency*, *77*, 654–669.

Campbell, B., & Jaynes, J. (1966). Reinstatement. *Psychological Review*, *73*, 478–480.

Campione, J. C., & Brown, A. L. (1977). Memory and metamemory development in educable retarded children. In R. V. Kail, Jr. & J. W. Hagen (Eds.), *Perspectives on the development of memory and cognition* (pp. 367–406). Hillsdale, NJ: Erlbaum.

Ceci, S. J. (1980). A developmental study of multiple encoding and its relationship to age related changes in free recall. *Child Development*, *51*, 892–895.

Ceci, S. J., & Howe, M. J. (1978). Age-related differences in free recall as a function of retrieval flexibility. *Journal of Experimental Child Psychology*, *26*, 432–442.

Cermak, S. L., Goldberg, J., Cermak, S., & Drake, C. (1980). The short-term memory ability of children with learning disabilities. *Journal of Learning Disabilities*, *13*, 25–29.

Chadwick, O., Rutter, M., Brown, G., Shaffer, D., & Traub, M. (1981). A prospective study of children with head injuries: II. Cognitive sequelae. *Psychological Medicine*, *11*, 49–61.

Chadwick, O., Rutter, M., Shaffer, D., & Shrout, P. E. (1981). A prospective study of children with head injuries: IV. Specific cognitive deficits. *Journal of Clinical Neuropsychology*, *3*, 101–120.

Chi, M. T. H. (1978). Knowledge structures and memory development. In R. Siegler (Ed.), *Children's thinking: What develops?* (pp. 73–96). Hillsdale, NJ: Erlbaum.

Cohen S., & deBettencourt, L. (1983). Teaching children to be independent learners: A step-by-step strategy. *Focus on Exceptional Children*, *16*, 1–12.

Cook, L. (1981). Misspelling analysis in dyslexia: Observation of developmental strategy shifts. *Bulletin of the Orton Society*, *31*, 123–134.

Crosson, B., Barco, P. P., Velozo, C. A., Bolesta, M. M., Cooper, P. V., Werts, D., & Brodbeck, T. C. (1989). Awareness and compensation in post-acute rehabilitation. *Journal of Head Trauma Rehabilitation*, *4*, 46–54.

DeLoache, J. (1985). Memory-based searching by very young children. In H. M. Wellman (Ed.), *Children's searching: The development of search skill and spatial representation* (pp. 151–183). Hillsdale, NJ: Erlbaum.

DeLoache, J., Cassidy, D., & Brown, A. (1985). Precursors of mnemonic strategies in very young children's memory. *Child Development*, *56*, 125–137.

Deshler, D. D., Alley, G. R., Warner, M. M., & Schumaker, J. B. (1981). Instructional practices for promoting skill acquisition and generalization in severely learning disabled adolescents. *Learning Disability Quarterly*, *4*, 415–421.

Douglas, V. I., Parry, P., Marton, P., & Garson, C. (1976). Assessment of a cognitive training program for hyperactive children. *Journal of Abnormal Child Psychology*, *4*, 389–410.

Englert, C. S., & Raphael, T. E. (1988). Constructing well-formed prose: Process, structure and metacognition in the instruction of expository writing. *Exceptional Children*, *54*, 513–520.

Entwisle, D. C. (1966). *The word association norms of young children*. Baltimore, MD: Johns Hopkins University Press.

Ewing, N., & Brecht, R. (1977). Diagnostic/prescriptive instruction: A recommendation of some issues. *Journal of Special Education*, *11*, 323–327.

Fagan, J. F. (1973). Infant's delayed recognition memory and forgetting. *Journal of Experimental Psychology*, *16*, 424–450.

Feuerstein, R. (1979). *The dynamic assessment of retarded performers: The learning potential device, theory, instruments, and techniques*. Baltimore, MD: University Park Press.

Feuerstein, R. (1980). *Instrumental enrichment: An intervention program for cognitive modifiability*. Baltimore, MD: University Park Press.

Flaro, L. (1987). The development and evaluation of a reading comprehension strategy with learning disabled students. *Reading Improvements*, *24*, 222–229.

Flavell, J. (1976). Metacognitive aspects of problem solving. In L. B. Resnick (Ed.), *The nature of intelligence* (pp. 231–235). Hillsdale, NJ: Erlbaum.

Flavell, J. (1979). Metacognition and cognitive monitoring: A new era of cognitive-developmental inquiry. *American Psychologist*, *34*, 907–911.

Flavell, J. (1985). *Cognitive development* (2nd ed.). Englewood Cliffs, NJ: Prentice-Hall.

Flavell, J. (1986). The development of children's knowledge about the appearance–reality distinction. *American Psychologist*, *41*, 418–425.

Forrest-Pressley, D. L., MacKinnon, G. E., & Waller, T. G. (Eds.) (1985a). *Metacognition, cognition, and human performance: Vol. 1. Theoretical perspectives*. Orlando, FL: Academic Press.

Forrest-Pressley, D. L., MacKinnon, G. E., & Waller, T. G. (Eds.) (1985b). *Metacognition, cognition, and human performance: Vol. 2. Instructional practices*. Orlando, FL: Academic Press.

Glidden, L. M., & Warner, D. A. (1985). Semantic processing and serial learning by EMR adolescents. *American Journal of Mental Deficiency*, *89*, 635–641.

Goldman, L. C., & Goldman, N. C. (1974). Problem-solving in the classroom: A model for sharing learning responsibility. *Educational Technology*, *9*, 53–58.

Goodland, J. (1983). *A place called school*. New York: McGraw-Hill.

Gordon, F., & Flavell, J. (1977). The development of intuitions about cognitive cueing. *Child Development*, *48*, 1027–1033.

Graham, S., & Freeman, S. (1986). Strategy training and teacher-vs.-student controlled study conditions: Effects on learning disabled students' spelling performance. *Learning Disabilities Quarterly*, *9*, 15–21.

Graham, S., & Harris, R. K. (1988). Instructional recommendations for teaching writing to exceptional students. *Exceptional Children*, *54*, 506–512.

Gresham, F. M. (1981). Social skills training with handicapped children. *Review of Educational Research*, *51*, 139–176.

Haarbauer-Krupa, J., Henry, K., Szekeres, S. F., & Ylvisaker, M. (1985). Cognitive rehabilitation therapy: Late stages of recovery. In M. Ylvisaker (Ed.), *Head injury rehabilitation: Children and adolescents* (pp. 311–343). Boston: College-Hill Press/Little, Brown.

Hagen, J., Jongeward, R., Jr., & Kail, R. (1975). Cognitive perspectives in the development of memory. In H. W. Reese (Ed.), *Advances in child development* (Vol 10, pp. 57–101). New York: Academic Press.

Hallahan, D. P., & Reeve, R. E. (1980). Selective attention and distractibility. In B. K. Keogh (Ed.), *Advances in special education: Vol. 1. Basic constructs and theoretical orientations* (pp. 141–181). Greenwich, CT: JAI Press.

Harris, K. R. (1982). Cognitive-behavior modification: Application with exceptional students. *Focus on Exceptional Children*, *15*, 1–16.

Hedberg, N., & Westby, C. (1991). *Narrative analysis manual*. Tuscon: Communication Skill Builders.

Henker, B., Whalen, C. K., & Hinshaw, S. P. (1980). The attributional contexts of cognitive intervention strategies. *Exceptional Education Quarterly*, *1*, 17–30.

Horowitz, L., Lampel, A., & Takanishi, R. (1969). The child's memory on unitized scenes. *Journal of Psychology*, *8*, 365–386.

Istominia, Z. M. (1977). The development of voluntary memory in preschool age children. *Soviet Psychology*, *13*, 5–64.

Jamison, P., & Shevitz, L. (1985). Rate: A reason to read. *Teaching Exceptional Children*, *18*, 46–50.

Jorgenson, C., Barrett, M., Huisingh, R., & Zachman, L. (1981). *The word test*. Moline, IL: Lingui Systems.

Kail, R. (1984). *The development of memory in children* (2nd ed). New York: Freeman.

Karoly, P. (1977). Behavioral self-management in children: Concepts, methods, issues, and directions. In M. Hersen, R. M. Eisler, & P. M. Miller (Eds.), *Progress in behavior modification* (Vol. 5, pp. 197–262). New York: Academic Press.

Karoly, P. (1984). Self-management problems in children. In E. J. Mash & L. G. Terdal (Eds.), *Behavioral assessment of childhood disorders* (pp. 79–126). New York: Guilford Press.

Kavale, K., & Mattson, P. (1983). "One jumped off the balance beam": Meta-analysis of perceptual-motor training. *Journal of Learning Disabilities*, *16*, 165–173.

Keeney, T., Cannizzo, S., & Flavell, J. (1967). Spontaneous and induced verbal rehearsal in a recall task. *Child Development*, *38*, 953–966.

Kellas, G., Ashcraft, M. H., & Johnson, N. S. (1973). Rehearsal processes in the short-term memory performance of mildly retarded adolescents. *American Journal of Mental Deficiency*, *77*, 670–679.

Keller, C. E., & Hallahan, D. P. (1987). *Learning disabilities: Issues and instructional interventions. What research says to the teacher.* Washington, DC: National Education Association Professional Library.

Kendall, P. C., & Finch, A. J. (1978). A cognitive-behavioral treatment for impulsivity: A group comparison study. *Journal of Consulting and Clinical Psychology*, *46*, 100–118.

Kendall, P. C., & Finch, A. J. (1979). Developing nonimpulsive behavior in children: Cognitive-behavioral strategies for self-control. In P. C. Kendall, & S. D. Hollon (Eds.), *Cognitive-behavioral interventions: Theory, research and procedures* (pp. 37–79). New York: Academic Press.

Keogh, B. K., & Margolis, J. (1976). Learn to labor and wait: Attentional problems of children with learning disorders. *Journal of Learning Disabilities*, *9*, 276–286.

Kirby, N. H., Nettlebeck, T., & Western, P. (1982). Locating information-processing deficits of mildly mentally retarded young adults. *American Journal of Mental Deficiency*, *87*, 338–343.

Klonoff, H., Low, M. D., & Clark, C. (1977). Head injuries in children: A prospective five year follow-up. *Journal of Neurology, Neurosurgery, and Psychiatry*, *40*, 1211–1219.

Kneedler, R. D., & Hallahan, D. P. (1981). Self-monitoring of on-task behavior with learning disabled children: Current studies and directions. *Exceptional Education Quarterly*, *2*, 73–82.

Kolb, B. (1989). Brain development, plasticity, and behavior. *American Psychologist*, *44*, 1203–1212.

Kreutzer, M. A., Leonard, C., & Flavell, J. H. (1975). An interview study of children's knowledge about memory. *Monographs of the Society for Research in Child Development*, *40*, Serial No. 159.

Lange, G. (1978). Organization-related processes in children's recall. In P. Ornstein (Ed.), *Memory development in children* (pp. 101–128). Hillsdale, NJ: Erlbaum.

Levin, H. S., Eisenberg, H. M., Wigg, N. R., & Kobayashi, K. (1982). Memory and intellectual ability after head injury in children and adolescents. *Neurosurgery*, *11*, 668–673.

Levine, H., & Langness, L. L. (1983). Everyday cognition among mildly mentally retarded adults: An ethnographic approach. *American Journal of Mental Deficiency*, *88*, 18–26.

Lezak, M. (1982). The problem of assessing executive functions. *International Journal of Psychology*, *17*, 281–297.

Lezak, M. (1987). Assessment for rehabilitation planning. In M. Meier, A. L. Benton, & L. Diller (Eds.), *Neuropsychological rehabilitation* (pp. 41–58). New York: Guilford Press.

Loper, A. (1980). Metacognitive development: Implication for cognitive training. *Exceptional Education Quarterly*, *1*, 1–8.

Lucariello, J., & Nelson, K. (1985). Slot-filler categories as memory organizers for young children. *Developmental Psychology*, *21*, 272–282.

Mandler, G. (1967). Organization and memory. In K. W. Spence & T. Spence (Eds.), *The psychology of learning and motivation: Vol 1. Advances in research and theory* (pp. 327–372). New York: Academic Press.

Markham, E. M. (1977). Realizing that you don't understand: A preliminary investigation. *Child Development*, *48*, 986–992.

Marzola, S. E. (1988). Interrogating the text: Questioning strategies designed to improve reading comprehension. *Reading, Writing, and Learning Disabilities*, *4*, 245–258.

McKinney, J. D., & Haskins, R. (1980). Cognitive training and the development of problem solving strategies. *Exceptional Education Quarterly*, *1*, 41–51.

McKinney, J. L., & Keen, P. G. W. (1976). How managers' minds work. *Harvard Business Review*, *52*, 14–21.

Meichenbaum, D. (1977). *Cognitive behavior modification: An integrative approach*. New York: Plenum.

Meichenbaum, D., & Asarnow, J. (1979). Cognitive-behavioral modification and metacognitive development: Implications for the classroom. In P. C. Kendall & S. D. Hollon (Eds.), *Cognitive-behavioral interventions: Theory, research, and procedures* (pp. 11–35). New York: Academic Press.

Meichenbaum, D., Burland, S., Gruson, L., & Cameron, R. (1985). Metacognitive assessment. In S. Yussen (Ed.), *The growth of reflection in children* (pp. 3–30). New York: Academic Press.

Meichenbaum, D., & Goodman, J. (1971). Training impulsive children to talk to themselves: A means of developing self-control. *Journal of Abnormal Psychology*, *77*, 115–126.

Meichenbaum, D., & Goodman, S. (1979). Clinical use of private speech and critical questions about it's study in natural settings. In G. Ziviu (Ed.), *The development of self-regulation through private speech* (pp. 115–126). New York: Wiley.

Merrill, E. C. (1985). Differences in semantic processing speed of mentally retarded and nonretarded persons. *American Journal of Mental Deficiency*, *90*, 71–80.

Messer, S. B. (1976). Reflection-impulsivity: A review. *Psychological Bulletin, 83*, 1026–1052.

Moely, B. (1977). Organization of memory. In R. Kail & J. Hagen (Eds.), *Perspectives on the development of memory and cognition* (pp. 203–236). Hillsdale, NJ: Erlbaum.

Moffat, N. (1984). Strategies of memory therapy. In B. Wilson & N. Moffat (Eds.), *Clinical management of memory problems* (pp. 63–88). Rockville, MD: Aspen Systems Corp.

Montague, M., & Bos, C. (1986). The effects of cognitive strategy training on verbal math problem-solving performance of L.D. adolescents. *Journal of Learning Disabilities, 19*, 26–33.

Myers, N., & Perlmutter, M. (1978). Memory in the years from two to five. In P. Ornstein (Ed.), *Memory development in children* (pp. 191–218). Hillsdale, NJ: Erlbaum.

Nelson, K. (1978). Semantic development and the development of semantic memory. In K. Nelson (Ed.), *Children's language* (Vol. 1, pp. 39–80). New York: Gardner Press.

Nelson, W. N. (1985). Teacher talk and child listening: Fostering a better match. In C. S. Simon (Ed.), *Communication skills and classroom success*. San Diego: College-Hill Press.

Nettlebeck T., & McLean, J. (1984). Mental retardation and inspection time: A two-stage model for sensory registration and central processing. *American Journal of Mental Deficiency, 89*, 83–90.

Ornstein, P., & Baker-Ward, L. (1983, April). *The development of mnemonic skill*. Paper presented at the meeting of the Society for Research in Child Development, Detroit, Michigan.

Palinscar, A. S. (1986). Metacognitive strategy instruction. *Exceptional Children, 53*, 118–124.

Pang, D. (1985). Pathophysiologic correlates of neurobehavioral syndromes following closed head injury. In M. Ylvisaker (Ed.), *Head injury rehabilitation: Children and adolescents* (pp. 3–70). Boston: College-Hill Press/Little, Brown.

Paris, S. G., & Oka, E. R. (1986). Self-regulated learning among exceptional children. *Exceptional Children, 53*, 103–108.

Patton, B. R., & Griffin, K. (1973). *Problem-solving group interaction*. New York: Harper & Row.

Pellegrino, J., & Ingram, A. (1978). *Processes, products and measures of memory organization* (Learning Research Development Center Report). Pittsburgh, PA: University of Pittsburgh.

Perlmutter, M., & Myers, N. A. (1979). Development of recall in 2-to-4 year old children. *Developmental Psychology, 15*, 73–83.

Perlmutter, M., & Ricks, M. (1979). Recall in preschool children. *Journal of Experimental Child Psychology, 27*, 423–436.

Petrey, S. (1977). Word association and the development of lexical memory. *Cognition, 5*, 57–71.

Pieper, E., & Deshler, D. D. (1985). Intervention considerations in mathematics for the learning disabled adolescent. *Focus on Learning Problems in Mathematics, 7*, 35–47.

Postman, L. (1964). Short-term memory and incidental learning. In A. W. Nelson (Ed.), *Categories of human learning* (pp. 145–201). New York: Academic Press.

Postman, L., & Kruesi, E. (1977). The influence of orienting tasks on the encoding and recall of words. *Journal of Verbal Learning and Verbal Behavior*, *2*, 353–369.

Pressley, M. (1979). Increasing children's self-control through cognitive interventions. *Review of Educational Research*, *49*, 319–370.

Pressley, M., & Brainerd, C. (1985). *Basic processes in memory development: Progress in cognitive development research*. New York: Springer-Verlag.

Pressley, M., Goodchild, F., Fleet, J., Zajchowski, R., & Evans, E. D. (1989). The challenges of classroom strategy instruction. *Elementary School Journal*, *89*, 301–342.

Pressley, M., & Levin, J. R. (Eds.) (1983a). *Cognitive strategy training: Educational applications*. New York: Springer-Verlag.

Pressley, M., & Levin, J. R. (Eds.) (1983b). *Cognitive strategy training: Psychological foundations*. New York: Springer-Verlag.

Prigatano, G. (1986). *Neuropsychological rehabilitation after brain injury*. Baltimore: Johns Hopkins University Press.

Raimondi, A. J., & Hirschauer, J. (1984). Head injury in the infant and toddler. *Child's Brain*, *11*, 12–35.

Ritter, K. (1978). The development of knowledge of an external retrieval cue strategy. *Child Development*, *49*, 1227–1230.

Ritter, K., Kaprove, B., Fitch, J., & Flavell, J. (1973). The development of retrieval strategies in young children. *Cognitive Psychology*, *5*, 310–332.

Rooney, K. J., & Hallahan, D. P. (1988). The effects of self-monitoring on adult behavior and student independence. *Learning Disabilities Research*, *3*, 88–93.

Rovee-Collier, C. (1984). The ontogeny of learning and memory in human infancy. In R. Kail & N. Spear (Eds.), *Comparative perspectives in the development of memory* (pp. 103–134). Hillsdale, NJ: Erlbaum.

Rummelhart, D. (1975). Notes on a schema for stories. In D. Brown & A. Collins (Eds.), *Representation and understanding. Studies on cognitive science* (pp. 237–272). New York: Academic Press.

Rutter, M. (1981). Psychological sequelae of brain damage in children. *American Journal of Psychiatry*, *138*, 1533–1544.

Rutter, M., Chadwick, O., Shaffer, D., & Brown, G. (1980). A prospective study of children with head injuries: I. Design and methods. *Psychological Medicine*, *10*, 633–646.

Ryan, E. B, Ledger, G. W., Short, E. J., & Weed, K. A. (1982). Promoting the use of active comprehension strategies by poor readers. *Topics in Learning and Learning Disabilities*, *2*, 53–60.

Sabatino, D. A., Miller, P. F., & Schmidt, C. (1981). Can intelligence be altered through cognitive training? *Journal of Special Education*, *15*, 125–144.

Salatas, H., & Flavell, J. H. (1976). Behavioral and metamnemonic indicators of strategic behaviors under instructions to remember in first grade. *Child Development*, *47*, 81–89.

Schacter, D. L., & Glisky, E. L. (1986). Memory remediation: Restoration, alleviation, and the acquisition of domain-specific knowledge. In B. Uzzell & Y. Gross (Eds.), *Clinical neuropsychology of intervention* (pp. 257–282). Boston: Martinus Nijhoff.

Schneider, W., & Pressley, M. (1989). *Memory development between 2 and 20*. New York: Springer-Verlag.

Seabaugh, G. O., & Schumaker, J. B. (1981). *The effects of self-regulation training on the academic productivity of LD and NLD adolescents* (Research Report No. 37). Lawrence: University of Kansas Institute for Research in Learning Disabilities.

Shapiro, E., & McCurdy, B. (1989). Effects of a taped word treatment on reading proficiency. *Exceptional Children*, *55*, 321–325.

Shields, J., & Heron, T. (1989). Teaching organizational skills to students with learning disabilities. *Teaching Exceptional Children*, *21*, 8–13.

Siegler, R. (1986). *Children's thinking*. Englewood Cliffs, NJ: Prentice-Hall.

Smirnov, A. (1973). *Problems in the psychology of memory*. New York: Plenum.

Sodian, B., Schneider, W., & Perlmutter, M. (1986). Recall, clustering and metamemory in young children. *Journal of Experimental Psychology*, *41*, 395–410.

Sophian, C. (1984). Developing search skills in infancy and early childhood. In C. Sophian (Ed.), *Origins of cognitive skills* (pp. 27–56). Hillsdale, NJ: Erlbaum.

Sophian, C., & Wellman, H. (1980). Selective information use in the development of search behavior. *Developmental Psychology*, *16*, 323–336.

Stein, N., & Glenn, C. (1979). An analysis of story comprehension in elementary school children. In R. Freedle (Ed.), *New directions in discourse processing* (pp. 53–120). Norwood, NJ: Ablex.

Szekeres, S. (1988). *Organization and recall in the young language impaired child*. Unpublished doctoral dissertation, University of Pittsburgh, Pittsburgh.

Taylor, B. M. (1982). Text structure and children's comprehension and memory for expository material. *Journal of Educational Psychology*, *74*, 323–340.

Thompson, R. W., & Hixson, P. K. (1984). Teaching parents to encourage independent problem solving in preschool-age children. *Language, Speech, and Hearing Services in the Schools*, *15*, 175–181.

Torgesen, J. (1985). Memory processes in reading disabled children. *Journal of Learning Disabilities*, *18*, 350–357.

Torgesen, J. (1988). Studies of children with learning disabilities who perform poorly on memory span tests. *Journal of Learning Disabilities*, *21*, 605–611.

Urbain, E. S., & Kendall, P. C. (1980). Review of Social-Cognitive Problem-Solving Interventions with Children. *Psychological Bulliten*, *88*, 109–143.

Van Reusen, T. (1987, May). *Training learning disabled adolescents to use a goal regulation strategy*. Paper presented at the PRISE Conference on Cognition and Metacognition, Pittsburgh, Pennsylvania.

Vellutino, F., & Scanlon, D. (1986). Experimental evidence for the effects of instructional bias on word identification. *Exceptional Children*, *52*, 145–156.

Weinstein, C., & Mayer, R. E. (1986). The teaching of learning strategies. In M. C. Wittrock (Ed.), *Handbook of research on teaching* (3rd ed., pp. 315–327). New York: Macmillan.

Wellman, H., Fabricius, W., & Sophian, C. (1985). The early development of planning. In H. M. Wellman (Ed.), *The development of search skill and spatial representation* (pp. 123–149). Hillsdale, NJ: Erlbaum.

Wellman, H. M., Ritter, R., & Flavell, J. H. (1975). Deliberate memory behavior in the delayed reactions of very young children. *Developmental Psychology*, *11*, 780–787.

Whitman, T. L. (1990). Self-regulation and mental retardation. *American Journal of Mental Retardation*, *94*, 347–362.

Wilson, B., & Moffat, N. (Eds.) (1984). *Clinical management of memory problems*. Rockville, MD: Aspen Systems Corp.
Wittrock, M. C. (1978). The cognitive movement in instruction. *Educational Psychologist*, *13*, 15–30.
Wong, B. (1986). Metacognition and special education: A review of a view. *Journal of Special Education*, *20*, 9–29.
Ylvisaker, M., & Szekeres, S. (1989). Metacognitive and executive impairments in head-injured children and adults. *Topics in Language Disorders*, *9*, 34–49.
Ylvisaker, M., Szekeres, S., Henry, K., Sullivan, D. M., & Wheeler, P. (1987). Topics in cognitive rehabilitation therapy. In M. Ylvisaker & E. M. R. Gobble (Eds.), *Community re-entry for head injured adults* (pp. 137–220). San Diego: College-Hill Press.

Appendix
Examples of Compensatory Strategies for Students with Cognitive Impairements[1]

I. Attention and concentration
   A. External aids
      1. Use a timer or alarm watch to focus attention for a specified period.
      2. Organize the work environment and eliminate distractions.
      3. Use a written or pictorial task plan with built-in rest periods and reinforcement; move a marker along to show progress.
      4. Place a symbol or picture card in an obvious place in the work areas as a reminder to maintain attention.
   B. Internal procedures
      1. Set increasingly demanding goals for self, including sustained work time.
      2. Self-instruct (e.g., "Am I wandering? What am I supposed to do? What should I be doing now?"). (Written cue cards may be needed during training period.)

II. Orientation (to time, place, person and event)
   A. External aids
      1. Use a log or journal book or tape recorder to record significant information and events of the day.

---

[1]From "Topics in Cognitive Rehabilitation Therapy" (pp. 216–220) by M. Ylvisaker, S. Szekeres, K. Henry, D. M. Sullivan, and P. Wheelero In *Community Re-entry for Head Injured Adults* edited by M. Ylvisaker and E. M. R. Gobble, 1987, San Diego: College-Hill Press. Copyright 1987 by College-Hill Press/Little, Brown. Reprinted with permission.

2. Refer to pictures of persons who are not readily identified (carry pictures attached to log book).
3. Use appointment book or daily schedule sheet.
4. Use alarm watch set for regular intervals.
5. Refer to maps or pictures for spatial orientation; make maps with landmarks.

B. Internal procedures
1. Select anchor points or events during the week and then attempt to reconstruct either previous or subsequent points in time (e.g., "My birthday was on Wednesday and that was yesterday, so this must be Thursday").
2. Request date, time, and similar information from others, when necessary.
3. Scan environment for landmarks.

III. Input control (amount, duration, complexity, rate, and interference).

A. Auditory
1. Give feedback to speaker (e.g., "Please slow down; speed up; break information into smaller 'chunks'; clarify").
2. Request repetition in another form (e.g., "Would you please write that down for me?").

B. Visual
1. Request longer viewing time or repeated viewings; request extra time for reading.
2. Cover parts of the page and look at exposed areas systematically, e.g., clockwise or left to right.
3. Use finger or index card to assist scanning and maintain place.
4. Use a symbol to mark right and left margins of written material or top and bottom segments as anchors in space.
5. Use large-print books or talking books.
6. Request a verbal description.
7. Remove an object from its setting to examine it; then return it to the original setting and view it again.
8. Place items in best visual field and eliminate visual distractors.
9. Turn head to compensate for field cut.

IV. Comprehension and memory process

A. Use self-questions (e.g., "Do I understand? Do I need to ask a question? How is this meaningful to me? How does this fit with what I know?"). Periodically look for gaps, misconceptions, or confusion (GMCs) by summarizing or explaining and checking back with speaker, a written source, or reference material.

B. Build "frames" or background for new information that is of particular significance or interest. Read summaries or general textbooks; ask knowledgeable persons about topic of special interest (a procedure in building frames).
C. Use a study guide for extended discourse material (e.g., SQ3R procedure: survey, question, read, recite, review).
D. Make charts and graphs of important relationships in textual material.
E. Use external memory aids (e.g., tape recorder, log book, notes, memos, written or pictured time lines).
F. Rehearse: covert or overt; auditory-vocal or motor (pantomime).
G. Organization: scan for or impose some order on incoming information.
H. Mnemonics: method of loci, rhymes, imagery (meaningful and novel associations).
I. Use diagrams or forms that facilitate deeper encoding of information and its subsequent retrieval.
J. Relate the information to personal life experiences and current knowledge. Use semantic knowledge of basic scripts (e.g., going to a restaurant, buying groceries) to help reconstruct previous events.
K. Project and describe situations in which target information will be needed or used.
L. At retrieval, reconstruct environment in which information was received.
M. Verbalize visual-spatial information (e.g., "*X* is to the left of *Y*"). Visualize verbal information in graphs, pictures, cartoons, or action-based imagery.
N. Keep items in designated places.

V. Word retrieval

A. Search lexical memory according to various categories and subcategories (e.g., person: family).
B. Describe the concept; circumlocute freely (talk about or around the subject).
C. Use gestures or signs.
D. Attempt to generate a sentence or use a carrier phrase.
E. Search letters or sounds of the alphabet (more effective in retrieving members of a limited category, such as names).
F. Describe perceptual attributes and semantic features of the concept.
G. Draw the item.
H. Attempt to write the word.

- I. Create an image of the object in a scene; then attempt to describe the scene.
- J. Attempt to retrieve the overlearned opposite.
- K. Free associate with image in mind.
- L. Associate a person's names with physical characteristics or a known person of the same name.

VI. Thought organization and verbal expression
- A. Use a structured thinking procedure.
- B. Use knowledge of scripts to generate real or imagined descriptions of experiences (narratives).
- C. Construct a time line to maintain appropriate sequence of events.
- D. Note topic in any conversation; self-question about the main point of expression; alert others before shifting from a topic abruptly.
- E. Watch others for feedback as to whether your words are confusing; watch facial expression, and so forth, or directly ask listeners, "Am I being clear?"
- F. Rehearse important comments or questions and listen to self.
- G. Set limits of time or allowable number of sentences in any one turn.

VII. Reasoning, problem solving, judgment
- A. Use a problem-solving guide.
- B. Use self-questioning for alternatives or consequences ("What else could I do?"; "What would happen if I did that?").
- C. Look at possible solutions from at least two different perspectives.
- D. Scan environment for cues as to appropriateness or inappropriateness of a behavior (e.g., facial expression of others; signs like "No Smoking"; formality versus informality of setting).
- E. Set specific times or places for behaviors that are appropriate only in specified situations.
- F. Actively envision situations to which successful procedures can be generalized.

VIII. Self-monitoring
- A. Use symbols or signs, placed in obvious places, or alarms that mean "pause" or "stop" or "Am I doing what I should be doing?"
- B. Use book or notebook with cards inserted at selected places with self-monitoring cues (e.g., "Summarize what you read").
- C. Pair specific self-instruction with the associated emotion (e.g., "Calm down" when angry).

IX. Task organization
   A. Use task organization checklist: materials, sequenced steps, time line, evaluation of results. Check each when completed.
   B. Prepare work space and assign space as task demands.

Epilogue

We have seen a varied blend of topics covered in this volume. In each case, the material was dealt with in a rigorous and integrative manner. Where appropriate, practical linkages were drawn. We were treated to examples of innovative work and "cutting edge" research, with new data graciously shared by many of the authors. For each advance or fresh insight that was discussed, important new questions were raised. All of this was most consistent with the spirit and stated objectives of the *Advances* series, as were outlined in the Preface.

Collectively, the works presented in this volume should give some idea of the diverse and exciting developments that are unfolding in the young but growing field of child neuropsychology. At one end, we have the kind of technical, highly specific, paradigmatic forms of investigation or application as exemplified in the works of Molfese (Chapter 1) and Hugdahl (Chapter 5). These dealt, respectively, with auditory evoked responses in newborns and with dichotic listening procedures. Both of these illustrated how knowledge regarding important neurodevelopmental parameters can be built in small but steady, stepwise increments, leading to substantial predictive power and potential clinical significance.

At the other end, the focus is wider, the questions are more complex and must be embedded within a biopsychosocial framework. This was exemplified in the work of both Taylor, Schatschneider, and Rich (Chapter 3) and Curley (Chapter 4) in which the determinants of developmental/behavioral outcomes associated with particular forms of brain disease or disorder were the focus of a broad-based yet rigorous analysis. In studying the effects of meningitis and childhood seizures, respectively, both investigations underscored the critical importance of evaluating those within the context of a carefully designated array of psychosocial factors. The Taylor et al. chapter went even further in providing an in-depth exposition of the many methodological issues inherent in studying the later effects of almost any type of early brain injury.

The topic of traumatic brain injury was covered from two perspectives. First, Fennell and Mickel (Chapter 2) provided a comprehensive overview of what is presently known regarding head trauma in children and adolescents—including its epidemiology, pathophysiology, and neurobehavioral effects. Next, Ylvisaker, Szekeres, and Hartwick (Chapter 6) examined head trauma from the standpoint of treatment, highlighting the rationale and essential components of a systematic, innovative, and ecologically-oriented approach to cognitive rehabilitation. Practical guidelines were offered, particularly with respect to educational interventions and specific modes of instruction indexed according to a careful consideration of the neuropsychological status of each child. This is an important and timely issue especially in view of the recent passage of U.S. Public Law 101–476, Individuals with Disabilities Education Act (IDEA), making traumatic brain injury a recognized category for special education services.

Much remains to be learned concerning developmental brain-behavior relationships, but the work to date has served to create a distinct base of knowledge that is sure to grow. Some outstanding examples were showcased in the present volume, but these were just a few of the many possibilities. There presently is work examining normal developmental parameters for functional processes such as attention. There are a host of investigations examining neuropsychological effects of childhood abnormalities as diverse as spina bifida, endocrine disorders, and cancer. There is also exemplary work dealing with assessment innovations, including the evaluation of infants, and with the development of empirically-derived programs of intervention for children with selected disabilities. These are some of the exciting areas that will be addressed in future volumes of *Advances in Child Neuropsychology*.

MICHAEL G. TRAMONTANA
STEPHEN R. HOOPER

Author Index

Subject Index